This book is dedicated to H. Allison Smith, Ph.D.
Best friend, wife, and mother of our wonderful children.

JDG

The authors would like to thank all of the publishers and authors for their permission to reproduce various tables and figures in this book. Special thanks to:

Advanced Technology Laboratories
The American College of Obstetricians and Gynecologists
The American College of Surgeons
The American Cancer Society
The American Society of Reproductive Medicine
The American Heart Association
The American Medical Association
Appleton & Lange
Blackwell Scientific Publishing
Churchill-Livingson
Dowden Publishing Company
Elsevier Scientific
The Female Patient
Hospital Practice Publishing
The Journal of Reproductive Medicine
Lippincott Williams Wilkins
Little, Brown and Company
McMahon Publishing Group
Medical Economics Company
Mosby Year Book
The New England Journal of Medicine
Oxford University Press
Springer Verlag
Thieme Medical Publishers
W.B. Saunders

Dr. Ricardo Asch
Dr. Emily Baker
Dr. Paul Barash
Dr. Arie Bergman
Dr. John Bonnar
Dr. Frank Chervenak
Dr. Steven Clark
Dr. Robert Creasy
Dr. Gary Cunningham
Dr. Richard Dorr
Dr. Arthur Fleischer
Dr. Mark Glezerman
Dr. Leonard Gomella
Dr. Neville Hacker
Dr. Vaclav Insler
Dr. Sidney Joel-Cohen
Dr. Howard Jones, III
Dr. Bruno Lunenfeld
Dr. Fred Miyazaki
Dr. Keith Moore
Dr. John Rock
Dr. James Scott
Dr. Phillip Sarrel
Dr. Lourdes Scheerer
Dr. Leonard Speroff
Dr. Alan Trounson
Dr. Richard Sweet
Dr. Frederick Zuspan
Dr. James Carter
Dr. David Halbert

Dr. Gordon extends his great appreciation to the following physicians for their contributions to this handbook since it was first published:

Alvaro Cuadros
LeRoy Heinrichs
Shirley Tom
Hal Holbrook
Emmet Lamb
David Grimes
Amin Milki
Linda Giudice
Katherine O'Hanlan
Giuliana Songster

Julie Neidich
Natalie Sohn
David Halbert
Clifford Goldstein
Jennifer Lublin
Laurie Swaim
Khoa Lai
James Carter
Usha Chitkara
Nelson Teng

Carl Levinson
John Arpels
Susan Ballagh
Michael Katz
Gretchen Flanagan
Ian Hardy
Babak Edraki
Dennis Siegler
Mary Lake Polan
Vicki Seltzer

Obstetrics Gynecology & Infertility

Handbook for Clinicians
Resident Survival Guide
5th Edition

John David Gordon, M.D.
Co-Director
Dominion Fertility
Arlington, Virginia

Associate Clinical Professor
Department of Obstetrics and Gynecology
The George Washington University

Jan T. Rydfors, M.D.
Clinical Assistant Professor
Department of Gynecology and Obstetrics
Stanford University Medical Center

Maurice L. Druzin, M.D.
Professor of Gynecology and Obstetrics
Director of Obstetrics
Stanford University Medical Center

Yona Tadir, M.D.
Professor of Obstetrics and Gynecology
Medical Director, Beckman Laser Institute
and Medical Clinic
University of California, Irvine

Technical and Computer Support:
Bill Gillespie
Director of Computer Operations
Department of Gynecology and Obstetrics
Stanford University Medical Center

Scrub Hill Press, Inc.
46 S. Glebe Road, Suite 301
Arlington, VA 22204
(301) 469-8854

ISBN 0-9645467-6-0

The opinions expressed in this book represent a broad range of opinions including those of the full-time and volunteer clinical faculty of the Department of Gynecology and Obstetrics at Stanford University. These opinions are not meant to represent a "standard of care" or a "protocol" but rather a guide to common clinical conditions. Use of these guidelines are obviously influenced by local factors, varying clinical circumstances, and honest differences of opinion.

The indications and dosages of all drugs in this book have been recommended in the medical literature and conform to the practices of the general medical community. The medications described do not necessarily have specific approval by the Food and Drug Administration for use in the diseases and dosages for which they are recommended. The package insert for each drug should be consulted for use and dosage as approved by the FDA. Because standards for usage change, it is advisable to keep abreast of revised recommendations, particularily those concerning new drugs.

Publisher: Scrub Hill Press, Inc.
Senior Editor: John David Gordon, MD
Editorial Assistance: Bill Todd, Bow Communications
Cover design: Christopher Carbone

For Additional Copies and Price List Contact:
John David Gordon, MD
Scrub Hill Press, Inc.
46 South Glebe Road, Suite 301
Arlington, VA 22204
Phone/Fax (301) 469-8854
e-mail: johndavidgordon@erols.com

First Edition - July 1991
Second Edition - February 1993
Third Edition - September 1993
Fourth Edition - January 1995
Revised Fourth Edition- October 1997

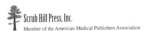

Scrub Hill Press, Inc.
Member of the American Medical Publishers Association

CONTENTS

PRIMARY CARE

OBSTETRICS

CONTENTS

CONTENTS

BREAST DISEASE

GYN-ONCOLOGY

⊃NTENTS

ENDOCRINOLOGY

INFERTILITY

ANATOMY

MICROBIOLOGY

CONTENTS

ᴏREWORD

This manual is dedicated to the Stanford Ob/Gyn residency. Written both by and for Stanford residents, it was initially developed as an introduction to the Ob/Gyn residency at Stanford to help new PGY-I residents with standard clinical protocols, important telephone numbers, and practical information on how to survive. Over the past three editions, the manual has been expanded to include clinical information beyond the algorithms of general obstetrics and gynecology. More complete information on the subspecialties of maternal-fetal medicine, reproductive endocrinology, and gyn-oncology has been included, as well as a broad base of general medical information which reflects the changing emphasis of Ob/Gyn as it expands to include primary care for women.

Although some of the specifics included in the manual have changed and more information has been added, its basic goal is still to provide a concise, easy-to-use, and immediately available handbook of information to make your life as a resident easier. All Ob/Gyn residencies are stressful and action-oriented with the requirement to absorb a tremendous amount of information in a short time. We hope that this manual will provide you with information which is useful for immediate patient care and provides a basis of practical knowledge upon which to build a career in obstetrics and gynecology using many other sources of information including books, journals, conferences, rounds, and practical teaching from your attendings.

Mary Lake Polan, M.D., Ph.D.
Professor and Chairman
Department of Gynecology and Obstetrics
Stanford University School of Medicine

PREFACE

This handbook was initially designed by residents for residents in an attempt to ease the transition between medical school and internship. It has proved to be a useful pocket reference for many of us, but please remember that the contents of this book are meant to be used as an aid in obstetrical and gynecologic decision making. It is not designed to serve as a replacement for traditional textbooks.

Since this handbook was initially published 10 years ago, I remain grateful to all of the residents, fellows, and physicians with whom I have worked for their understanding and emotional support especially Henry, Dave, Mack, Pamela and Laurie at UT-Houston; Yasser, Ron, Jean, Dennis, Debbie, Thomas and Anjali at Stanford; Russell, Collin and Jan at UCSF.

Sincere thanks to Bill Todd for his outstanding editorial assistance. Without the endless patience and technical support of Bill Gillespie, publication of the book would not have been possible. For the computer crowd, this entire book was produced on a Macintosh computer using Adobe PageMaker 6.52.

Over the past 10 years a number of people have contributed to the success of this project and the formation of Scrub Hill Press, Inc. In particular, I would like to thank Becky Morris (and the staff of Stanford Publication Services), Jean Williams, Randy Winn, Donna Troyna, J. Peter Shearer, John Hardee, Fred Peterson, Robert Howard, Chris Carbone, and Dan Poyner.

My co-editors have remained enthusiastic and supportive over the years. Dr. Yona Tadir's contributions significantly improved the quality of the Fourth Edition and I am grateful to him for all of his hard work. Dr. Jan Rydfors has been a part of this project since it was conceived and I appreciate his outstanding contribution to the content of the guide. Finally, Dr. Maurice Druzin has been my mentor since residency at Stanford and although we live on opposite coasts I know that his wisdom and sage advice are always just a phone call away.

It has been my fortune to have trained under a series of outstanding Department Chairman: Dr. Charles Hammond, Dr. Robert Creasy, Dr. Mary Lake Polan, and Dr. Robert Jaffe. I am forever indebted to them for their patience in dealing with the author of this book. In addition, I would like to thank Dr. Michael DiMattina who has remained supportive of my publishing activities during the past few years of working side-by-side at Dominion Fertility & Endocrinology.

This project would not have been possible without the generous financial and emotional support of my parents, Dr. and Mrs. Edward T. Gordon.

Finally, this Fifth Edition of the handbook remains dedicated to H. Allison Smith, loving wife, mother of our children, and best friend for all of her support through medical school, two internships, residency, fellowship training and beyond.

John David Gordon, M.D.
Co-Director
Dominion Fertility & Endocrinology

Clinical Associate Professor
The George Washington University
Department of Obstetrics and Gynecology

HEALTH MAINTENANCE

Controversy exists regarding screening and immunizations for adults. The following guidelines have been generated by the Palo Alto Medical Foundation (a large multi-specialty medical foundation associated with Stanford University Medical Center). The following guidelines are intended as minimal screening recommendations for patients considered to be at average risk. Physicians should take into consideration the standard of care within their own communities.

Screening Test	Comments
Cholesterol	Non-fasting total cholesterol every 5 years; HDL/LDL per physician discretion
Rectal exam	Yearly > 50 yr (> 40 yr per physician discretion)
Occult blood in stool	Yearly > 50 yr
Sigmoidoscopy	Every 5 years > 50 yr
Colonoscopy	Highest risk population (ulcerative colitis, polyposis, > 40 yr and 1st degree relative with colon cancer)
Pap smear	Yearly (less frequent per physician discretion after 3 normal tests)
Chlamydia	High risk population
Breast exam	Yearly
Pelvic exam	Yearly, even if Pap deferred, as long as uterus present
Mammography	Every 2 years > 40 yr; Yearly > 50 yr (This recommendation is controversial)
dT (Tetanus vaccine)	Every 10 years
Measles vaccine	Booster x1 if born after 1956
Rubella vaccine	Potentially childbearing female without proof of immunity or booster
Influenza vaccine	a) Yearly > 65 yr b) Any age with high risk medical problem (cardiac, renal, hematologic, pulmonary disease, etc.) c) Residents of chronic care facilities d) Health care providers for high risk patients e) Household contacts of high risk patients
Pneumococcus vaccine	a) Once > 65 b) Any age with high risk problem as above
PPD (TB skin test)	a) Household or close contact with person with infectious TB, HIV infection, or CXR consistent with old healed TB (Positive test is > 5 mm induration) b) High risk individuals: immigrants from endemic areas, alcoholics, IV drug users, residents of chronic care facilities c) Low risk adults: Not recommended (Positive test is > 15 mm induration)
Hepatitis B	a) Surface antigen screening of endemic populations: natives of Asia, Southeast Asia, Pacific Islands, Arctic, India, sub-Sahara Africa, Haiti b) If positive, screen and vaccinate household contacts c) Hepatoma screening recommendations deferred pending further information d) Consider vaccination in IV drug users, health professionals, chronic blood product recipients

PRIMARY CARE

NUTRITION

Nutrient	Nonpregnant	Pregnant	Lactating	Dietary Source
Energy	2200 kcal	2500 kcal	2800 kcal	Protein, fat, carbohydrate
Protein	50 g	60 g	65 g	Meats, fish, poultry, dairy
Fat-Soluble Vitamins				
Vitamin A*	800 µg	800 µg	1300 µg	Green leafy or dark yellow vegetables, liver, milk
Vitamin D§	5 µg	10 µg	10 µg	Fortified dairy products, fish liver oil, sunshine
Vitamin E¥	8 mg	10 mg	12 mg	Vegetable oils, whole-grain cereals, nuts, leafy vegetables
Vitamin K	65 µg	65 µg	65 µg	Green vegetables, tomatoes, dairy products
Water-Soluble Vitamins				
Vitamin C	60 mg	70 mg	95 mg	Citrus fruits, strawberries, broccoli, tomatoes
Thiamine (B1)	1.1 mg	1.5 g	1.6 mg	Enriched grains, legumes, pork
Riboflavin (B2)	1.3 mg	1.6 mg	1.8 mg	Meats, liver, grains
Niacin φ	15 mg	17 mg	20 mg	Meats, nuts, legumes
Vitamin B6	1.6 mg	2.2 mg	2.1 mg	Poultry, fish, liver, eggs
Folate	180 µg	400 µg	280 µg	Leafy vegetables, orange juice, strawberries, liver, legumes
Vitamin B12	2 µg	2.2 µg	2.6 µg	Animal proteins
Minerals				
Calcium	800 mg	1200 mg	1200 mg	Dairy products, collard, kale, mustard and turnip greens
Phosphorus	800 mg	1200 mg	1200 mg	Meats
Magnesium	280 mg	320 mg	355 mg	Seafood, legumes, grains
Iron	15 mg	30 mg	15 mg	Meats, eggs, grains, dried beans, prune juice
Zinc	12 mg	15 mg	19 mg	Meats, seafood, eggs
Iodine	150 µg	175 µg	200 µg	Iodized salt, seafood
Selenium	55 µg	65 µg	75 µg	Seafood, liver, meats

* Retinol equivalents (RE) 1 retinol equivalent = 1 µg retinol or 6 µg β-carotene
§ As cholecalciferol. 10 µg cholecalciferol = 400 IU Vitamin D
¥ α-Tocopherol equivalents (TE) 1 mg D-α-tocopherol= 1 α-TE
φ Niacin equivalent (NE) = 1 mg of niacin or 60 mg of dietary tryptophan

Source: Kochenour NK. Normal pregnancy and prenatal care. In: Scott JR, DiSaia PD, Hammond CB, Spellacy WN, ed. *Danforth's Obstetrics and Gynecology.* 7th ed. Philadelphia: Lippincott, 1994. Reproduced with the permission of the publisher.

BODY MASS INDEX

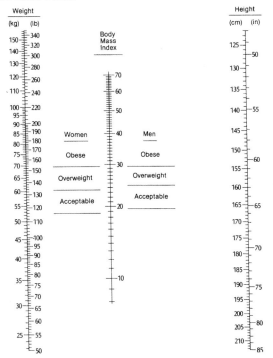

Source: Speroff L, Glass RH, Kase NG. Obesity. In: *Clinical Gynecologic Endocrinology and Infertility*. 6th ed. Philadelphia: Lippincott Williams & Wilkins, 1999. Reproduced with the permission of the publisher.

PRIMARY CARE

HYPERCHOLESTEROLEMIA TREATMENT
Reproduced from the National Cholesterol Education Program Expert Panel on Detection, Evaluation and Treatment of High Blood Cholesterol in Adults (Adult Treatment Panel III).

ATP III Recommendations
Step 1: Determine lipoprotein levels - obtain complete lipoprotein profile after 9- to 12- hour fast.

LDL Cholesterol - Primary Target of Therapy	
<100	Optimal
100-129	Near optimal/above optimal
130-159	Borderline high
160-189	High
190	Very high
Total Cholesterol	
< 200	Desirable
200-239	Borderline high
240	High
HDL Cholesterol	
<40	Low
60	High

Step 2: Identify presence of clinical atherosclerotic disease that confers high risk for coronary heart disease (CHD) events (CHD risk equivalent):
- Clinical CHD
- Symptomatic carotid artery disease
- Peripheral artery disease
- Abdominal aortic aneurysm

Step 3: Determine the presence of major risk factors (other than LDL):
- Cigarette smoking
- Hypertension (BP ≥140/90 mmHg or on antihypertensive therapy)
- Low HDL cholesterol (<40 mg/dL)*
- Family history of premature CHD (male first degree relative <55 years, female first degree relative <65 years)
- Age (men≥45 years; women ≥55 years)

*HDL cholesterol ≥60 mg/dL counts as "negative" risk factor, its presence removes one risk factor from total count

NOTE: in ATP III, diabetes is regarded as a CHD risk equivalent.

Step 4: If 2+ risk factors (other than LDL) are present without CHD or CHD risk equivalent, assess 10 year (short-term) CHD risk (see Framingham tables). Three levels of 10-year risk:
- >20% - CHD risk equivalent
- 10-20%
- <10%

HYPERCHOLESTEROLEMIA TREATMENT (CONT.)
ATP III Recommendations (cont.)

Step 5: Determine risk category:
- Establish LDL goal of therapy
- Determine need for therapeutic lifestyle changes (TLC)
- Determine level for drug consideration

Risk Category	LDL Goal	LDL Level at Which to Initiate Therapeutic Lifestyle Changes (TLC)	LDL Level at Which to Consider Drug Therapy
CHD or CHD Risk Equivalents (10-year risk >20%)	<100 mg/dL	100 mg/dL	>130 mg/dL (100-129 mg/dL:drug optional)*
2+ Risk Factors	<130 mg/dL	130 mg/dL	10-year risk 10-20%: 130 mg/dL 10-year risk <10%: 160 mg/dL
0-1 Risk Factors ¥	<160 mg/dL	160 mg/dL	190 mg/dL (160-189 mg/dL: LDL-lowering drug optional)

* Some authorities recommend use of LDL-lowering drugs in this category if an LDL cholesterol <100 mg/dL cannot be achieved by therapeutic lifestyle changes. Others prefer use of drugs that primarily modify triglycerides and HDL, e.g., nicotinic acid or fibrate. Clinical judgement also may call for deferring drug therapy in this subcategory.

¥ Almost all people with 0-1 risk factors have a 10-year risk <10%, thus 10-year risk assessment in people with 0-1 risk factors is not necessary.

Step 6: Initiate therapeutic lifestyle changes (TLC) if LDL is above goal.
TLC Features
- TLC Diet
  - Saturated fat <7% of calories, cholesterol <200 mg/dL
  - Consider increased viscous (soluble) fiber (10-25 g/day) and plant stanols/sterols (2g/day) as therapeutic options to enhance LDL lowering
- Weight management
- Increased physical activity

Step 7: Consider adding drug therapy if LDL exceeds levels shown in Step 5 table:
- Consider drug simultaneously with TLC for CHD and CHD equivalents
- Consider adding drug to TLC after 3 months for other risk categories

HYPERCHOLESTEROLEMIA TREATMENT (CONT.)
ATP III Recommendations (cont)
Step 7 (cont)

Class of Drug	Typical Daily Dose	Lipid/Lipoprotein Effects	Side Effects	Contraindications
HMG CoA reductase inhibitors (" statins ")				
Atorvastatin (Lipitor)	10-80 mg	LDL-C ↓18-55%	Myopathy	Absolute
Lovastatin (Mevacor)	20 mg	HDL-C ↑ 5-15%	Increased liver	• Active or chronic liver
Simvastatin (Zocor)	20-80 mg	TG ↓7-30%	enzymes	disease
Pravastatin (Pravachol)	20-40 mg			
Fluvastatin (Lescol)	20-80 mg			Relative
Cerivastatin	0.4-0.8 mg			• Concomitant use of certain drugs*
Bile acid sequestrants or resins				
Cholestyramine (Questran)	4-16 g	LDL-C ↓15-30%	Gastrointestinal	Absolute
Colestipol (Colestid)	5-20 g	HDL-C ↑ 3-5%	distress	• dysbetalipoproteinemia
Colesevelam	2.6-3.8 g	TG No change	Constipation	• TG>400 mg/dL
			Decreased absorption of	Relative
			other drugs	• TG>200 mg/dL
Nicotinic acid				
Niacin (Niacor)	1 g tid	LDL-C ↓5-25%	Flushing	Absolute
		HDL-C ↑ 15-35%	Hyperglycemia	• Chronic liver disease
		TG ↓20-50%	Hyperuricemia (or gout)	• Severe gout
			Upper GI distress	Relative
			Hepatotoxicity	• Diabetes
				• Hyperuricemia
				• Peptic ulcer disease
Fibric acis				
Gemfibrozil (Lopid)	600 mg bid	LDL-C ↓5-20%	Dyspepsia	Absolute
Clofibrate (Atromid)	1 g bid	(may be increased in	Gallstones	• Severe renal disease
Fenofibrate	200 mg	patients with high TG)	Myopathy	• Severe hepatic disease
		HDL-C ↑ 10-20%		
		TG ↓20-50%		

* Cyclosporine, macrolide antibiotics, various anti-fungal agents, and cytochrome P-450 inhibitors (fibrates and niacin should be used with appropriate caution).

Step 8: Identify metabolic syndrome and treat, if present, after 3 months of TLC.

Treatment of the metabolic syndrome
• Treat underlying causes (overweight/obesity and physical inactivity):
- Intensify weight management
- Increase physical activity
• Treat lipid and non-lipid risk factors if they persist despite these lifestyle therapies:
- Treat hypertension
- Use aspirin for CHD patients to reduce prothrombotic state
- Treat elevated triglycerides and/or low HDL (as shown in Step 9)

HYPERCHOLESTEROLEMIA TREATMENT (CONT.)

ATP III Recommendations (cont)

Clinical identification of the Metabolic Syndrome

Risk Factor	Defining Level
Abdominal obesity*	Waist circumference
Men	>102 cm (>40 in)
Women	>88 cm (>35 in)
Triglycerides	150 mg/dL
HDL cholesterol	
Men	<40 mg/dL
Women	<50 mg/dL
Blood pressure	130/85 mmHg
Fasting glucose	110 mg/dL

* Overweight and obesity are associated with insulin resistance and the metabolic syndrome. However, the presence of abdominal obesity is more highly correlated with the metabolic risk factors than is an elevated body mass index (BMI). Therefore the simple measure of waist circumference is recommended to identify the body weight component of the metabolic syndrome.

Step 9: Treat elevated triglycerides or isolated low HDL

Treatment of elevated triglycerides (≥150 mg/dL)
- Primary aim of therapy is to reach LDL goal.
- Intensify weight management
- Increase physical activity.
- If triglycerides are ≥200 mg/dL after LDL goal is reached, set secondary goal for non-HDL cholesterol (total -HDL) 30 mg/dL higher than LDL goal

If triglycerides are 200-499 mg/dL after LDL goal is reached, consider adding drug if needed to reach non-HDL goal:
- Intensify therpy with LDL-lowering drug, or
- Add nicotinic acid or fibrate to further lower VLDL

If triglycerides are ≥500 mg/dL, first lower triglycerides to prevent pancreatitis:
- Very low fat diet (≤15% of calories from fat)
- Weight management and physical activity
- Fibrate or nicotinic acid
- When triglycerides are <500 mg/dL, turn to LDL-lowering therapy

Treatment of low HDL cholesterol (≤40 mg/dL)
- First reach LDL goal
- Intensify weight management and increase physical activity
- If triglycerides are 200-499 mg/dL, achieve non-HDL goal.
- If triglycerides are <200 mg/dL (isolated low HDL) in CHD or CHD equivalent, consider nicotinic acid or fibrate.

PRIMARY CARE

HYPERTENSION
JNC VI Risk Stratification and Treatment Recommendations
- Determine blood pressure stage
- Determine risk group by major risk factors and TOD/CCD
- Determine treatment recommendations (by using table below)
- Determine goal blood pressure
- Refer to specific treatment recommendations

Major Risk Factors
- Smoking
- Dyslipidemia
- Diabetes mellitus
- Age >60 years
- Male gender or postmenopausal female
- Family history of first degree relative < 55 years (men) or <65 years (women)

Target Organ Damage/Clinical Cardiovascular Disease (TOD/CCD)
- Heart diseases
  - Left ventricular hypertrophy
  - Angina or prior myocardial infarction
  - Prior CABG
  - Heart failure
- Stroke or TIA
- Nephropathy
- Peripheral artery disease
- Hypertensive retinopathy

Blood Pressure Stages (mm Hg)	Risk Group A No major risk factors No TOD/CCD	Risk Group B At least one major risk factor not including diabetes No TOD/CCD	Risk Group C TOD/CCD and/or diabetes with or without other risk factors
High-normal (130-139/85-89)	Lifestyle modification	Lifestyle modification	Drug therapy for those with heart failure, renal insufficiency or diabetes. Lifestyle modification
Stage 1 (140-159/90-99)	Lifestyle modification (up to 12 months)	Lifestyle modification (up to 6 months) For patients with multiple risk factors, clinicians should consider drugs as initial therapy plus lifestyle modifications.	Drug therapy Lifestyle modification
Stages 2 and 3 (≥ 160/≥ 100)	Drug therapy Lifestyle modification	Drug therapy Lifestyle modification	Drug therapy Lifestyle modification

Goal Blood Pressure

<140/90 mm Hg	Uncomplicated hypertension, Risk Group A, Risk Group B, Risk Group C except for the following:
<130/85 mm Hg	Diabetes; renal failure; heart failure
<125/75 mm Hg	Renal failure with proteinuria >1 gram/24 hours

Source: *The Sixth Report of the Joint National Committee on Prevention, Detection, Evaluation, and Treatment of High Blood Pressure.* Arch Intern Med 1997;157:2413-2446. NIH Publication No. 98-4080.

PHARMACOLOGIC MANAGEMENT OF HYPERTENSION
JNC VI Treatment Recommendations

Initial Drug Choices
- Start with a low dose of a long-acting once-daily drug and titrate dose
- Low-dose combinations may be appropriate

Uncomplicated Hypertension	Compelling Indications		Specific Indications for the Following Drugs
Diuretics Beta-blockers	Diabetes type 1 (IDDM)	Start with ACE inhibitor if proteinuria is present	(See Table 9 in JNC VI for specific indications) ACE inhibitors Angiotensin II receptor blockers Alpha-blockers Alpha-beta-blockers Beta-blockers Calcium antagonists Diuretics
	Heart failure	Start with ACE inhibitor or diuretic	
	Myocardial infarction	Beta-blocker (non-ISA) after MI; ACE inhibitor for LV dysfunction after MI	
	Isolated systolic hypertension (older patients)	Diuretics (preferred) or calcium antagonists (long-acting DHP)	

Source: *The Sixth Report of the Joint National Committee on Prevention, Detection, Evaluation, and Treatment of High Blood Pressure. Arch Intern Med* 1997;157:2413-2446. NIH Publication No. 98-4080.

Class and Medication	Normal Daily Dosage in mg/d (interval)	Dispensing Unit (mg)
Angiotensin-converting enzyme (ACE) inhibitors		
Captopril	75-450 (tid)	12.5, 25, 50, 100
Enalapril	5-40 (qd, bid)	2.5, 5, 10, 20
Calcium channel blockers		
Nifedipine (sustained release)	30-90 (qd)	30, 60, 90
Diltiazem (sustained release)	120-240 (qd)	60, 90, 120
Verapamil (sustained release)	120-480 (qd, bid)	120, 180, 240
Alpha blockers		
Prazosin	2-20 (bid, tid, qid)	1, 2, 5
Terazosin	1-20 (qd)	1, 2, 5, 10
Mixed alpha and beta blockers		
Labetalol	200-800 (bid)	100, 200, 300
Diuretics		
Hydrochlorothiazide	12.5-50 (qd)	25, 50
Furosemide (loop diuretic)	20-1,000 (qd-bid)	20, 40, 80
Triamterene (potassium-sparing)	50-100 (bid)	50, 100
Beta blockers		
Propranolol (lipid soluble)	60-160 (qd)	60, 80, 120, 160
Atenolol (water soluble)	50-100 (qd)	50, 100
Central agents		
Methyldopa	250-2,000 (bid)	125, 250, 500

Source: Management of Medical Disorders. *Primary and Preventive Care: A Primer for Obstetricians and Gynecologists,* American College of Obstetricians and Gynecologists, Washington, DC, 1994. Reproduced with permission.

PRIMARY CARE

DEPRESSION

Fast Facts
• major depressive episode affects 20 million American adults yearly
• twice as frequent in women
• mean age of onset: 40 years old
• only 20-25% of patients receive appropriate care

Predisposing Factors for Women
• childhood loss (e.g. death or illness of a parent)
• physical or sexual abuse (domestic violence)
• socioeconomic deprivation
• genetic predisposition
• perinatal loss, infertility, miscarriage
• menopause

Diagnosis
• patients may present with mood disorder or somatic complaints
  • chronic, clinically unconfirmed vaginitis
  • idiopathic vulvodynia
  • chronic vaginal, pelvic pain
  • severe, incapacitating PMS
  • dysmenorrhea, dyspareunia, sexual dysfunction

DSM-IV Criteria for Major Depressive Episode

Five or more of the following symptoms have been present during the same 2-week period and represent a change from previous functioning; at least one of the symptoms is either (1) depressed mood or (2) loss of interest or pleasure.

Note: Do not include symptoms that are clearly due to a general medical condition, or mood-incongruent delusions or hallucinations.

1. Depressed mood most of the day, nearly every day, as indicated by either subjective report (e.g., feels sad or empty) or observation made by others (e.g., appears tearful).
2. Markedly diminished interest or pleasure in all, or almost all, activities most of the day, nearly every day (as indicated by either subjective account or observation made by others).
3. Significant weight loss when not dieting or weight gain (e.g., a change of more than 5% of body weight in a month), or decrease or increase in appetite nearly every day.
4. Insomnia or hypersomnia nearly every day
5. Psychomotor agitation or retardation nearly every day (observable by others, not merely subjective feelings of restlessness or being slowed down).
6. Fatigue or loss of energy nearly every day.
7. Feelings of worthlessness or excessive or inappropriate guilt (which may be delusional) nearly every day (not merely self-reproach or guilt about being sick).
8. Diminished ability to think or concentrate, or indecisiveness, nearly every day (either by subjective account or as observed by others).
9. Recurrent thoughts of death (not just fear of dying), recurrent suicidal ideation without a specific plan, or a suicide attempt or a specific plan for committing suicide.

MAJOR DEPRESSIVE AND OTHER PSYCHIATRIC DISORDERS

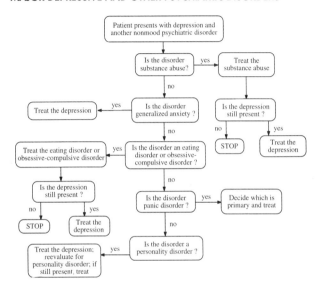

When depression is treated, the anxiety disorder should resolve as well.
Choose medications known to be effective for both the depression and the other psychiatric disorder.
Primary is the most severe, the longest standing by history, or the one that runs in the patient's family.
In certain cases, both major depression and substance abuse may require simultaneous treatment.

Source: Depression Guideline Panel. *Depression in Primary Care: Detection, Diagnosis, and Treatment.* Quick Reference Guide for Clinicians, Number 5, Rockville, MD. US Department of Health and Human Services, Public Health Service, Agency for Health Care Policy and Research. AHCPR Publication 93-0552. April, 1993.

PRIMARY CARE

OVERVIEW OF TREATMENT FOR DEPRESSION

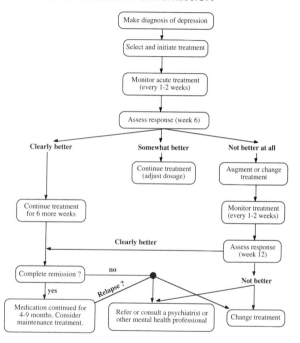

Source: Depression Guideline Panel. *Depression in Primary Care: Detection, Diagnosis, and Treatment.* Quick Reference Guide for Clinicians, Number 5, Rockville, MD. US Department of Health and Human Services, Public Health Service, Agency for Health Care Policy and Research. AHCPR Publication 93-0552. April, 1993.

SIX-WEEK EVALUATION: PARTIAL OR NONRESPONDERS TO MEDICATION

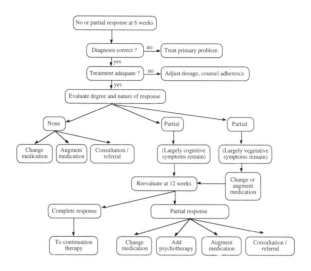

No response - patient is nearly as symptomatic as at pretreatment
Partial response - patient is clearly better than at pretreatment, but still has significant symptoms. Consultation or referral may be valuable before proceeding further.

Suggestions for management are based on some indirectly relevant studies, logic, and clinical experience.

Source: Depression Guideline Panel. *Depression in Primary Care: Detection, Diagnosis, and Treatment.* Quick Reference Guide for Clinicians, Number 5, Rockville, MD. US Department of Health and Human Services, Public Health Service, Agency for Health Care Policy and Research. AHCPR Publication 93-0552. April, 1993.

PRIMARY CARE

TREATMENT OPTIONS FOR DEPRESSION
Medication
- over 50% of patients will experience marked improvement or complete remission
- considerations for treatment with medication as acute phase therapy include:
  - more severe symptoms
  - chronicity
  - recurrent episodes (≥ 2 prior episodes)
  - presence of psychotic features (hallucinations or delusions)
  - presence of melancholic symptoms
  - family history of depression
  - prior response to medication treatment
  - incomplete response to psychotherapy alone
  - patient preference

Psychotherapy
- effective in mild to moderate depression
- usually cognitive, interpersonal or behavioral
- considerations for acute phase treatment with psychotherapy include:
  - less severe depression
  - less recurrent, chronic or disabling depression
  - absence of psychotic symptoms
  - prior positive response to psychotherapy
  - incomplete response to medication alone
  - chronic psychosocial problems
  - medication contraindicated or refused
  - patient preference

Combined Treatment
- should be considered in various situations including:
  - more severe depression
  - recurrent depression with poor interepisode recovery
  - incomplete therapeutic response to either psychotherapy or medication alone
  - evidence of a significant personality disorder
  - patient preference

Source: Depression Guideline Panel. *Depression in Primary Care: Detection, Diagnosis, and Treatment.* Quick Reference Guide for Clinicians, Number 5. Rockville, MD. US Department of Health and Human Services, Public Health Service, Agency for Health Care Policy and Research. AHCPR Publication 93-0552. April, 1993.

ANTIDEPRESSANT MEDICATIONS

Drug	Therapeutic Dosage Range (mg/day)	Potentially Fatal Drug Interactions
Tricyclics		
Amitriptyline (Elavil, Endep)	75-300	Antiarrhythmics, MAOI's
Clomipramine (Anafranil)	75-300	Antiarrhythmics, MAOI's
Desipramine (Norpramin, Pertofrane)	75-300	Antiarrhythmics, MAOI's
Doxepin (Adaptin, Sinequan)	75-300	Antiarrhythmics, MAOI's
Imipramine (Janimine, Tofranil)	75-300	Antiarrhythmics, MAOI's
Nortriptyline (Aventyl, Pamelor)	75-300	Antiarrhythmics, MAOI's
Protriptyline (Vivactil)	75-300	Antiarrhythmics, MAOI's
Trimipramine (Surmontil)	75-300	Antiarrhythmics, MAOI's
Heterocyclics		
Amoxapine (Asendin)	100-600	MAOI's
Bupropion (Wellbutrin, Zyban)	225-450	MAOI's (possibly)
Maprotiline (Ludiomil)	100-225	MAOI's
Trazodone (Desyrel)	150-600	
Selective Serotonin Reuptake Inhibitors (SSRI's)		
Fluoxetine (Prozac)	10-40	MAOI's
Paroxetine (Paxil)	20-50	MAOI's
Sertraline (Zoloft)	50-150	MAOI's
Monoamine Oxidase Inhibitors (MAOI's)		
Isocarboxazid (Marplan)	0-50	For all 3 MAOI's: vasoconstrictors, decongestants*, meperidine, and possibly other narcotics
Phenelzine (Nardil)	45-90	
Tranylcypromine (Parnate)	20-60	

* Including pseudoephedrine, phenylephrine, phenylpropanolamine, epinephrine, norepinephrine, and others.

PRIMARY CARE

SIDE EFFECTS OF ANTIDEPRESSANT MEDICATIONS

Drug	Anticholinergic	Drowsiness	Insomnia Agitation	Orthostatic Hypotension	Arrhythmias	GI Distress	Weight Gain (> 6 kg)
Amitriptyline (Elavil, Endep)	4+	4+	0	4+	3+	0	4+
Desipramine (Norpramin, Pertofrane)	1+	1+	1+	2+	2+	0	1+
Doxepin (Adaptin, Sinequan)	3+	4+	0	2+	2+	0	3+
Imipramine (Janimine, Tofranil)	3+	3+	1+	4+	3+	1+	3+
Nortriptyline (Aventyl, Pamelor)	1+	1+	0	2+	2+	0	1+
Protriptyline (Vivactil)	2+	1+	1+	2+	2+	0	0
Trimipramine (Surmontil)	1+	4+	0	2+	2+	0	3+
Amoxapine (Asendin)	2+	2+	2+	2+	3+	0	1+
Maprotiline (Ludiomil)	2+	4+	0	0	1+	0	2+
Trazodone (Desyrel)	0	4+	0	1+	1+	1+	1+
Bupropion (Wellbutrin)	0	0	2+	0	1+	1+	0
Fluoxetine (Prozac)	0	0	2+	0	0	3+	0
Paroxetine (Paxil)	0	0	2+	0	0	3+	0
Sertraline (Zoloft)	0	0	2+	0	0	3+	0
Monoamine Oxidase Inhibitors	1+	1+	2+	2+	0	1+	2+

* Anticholinergic side-effects: dry mouth, blurred vision, urinary hesitancy, constipation

```
0 = absent or rare
1+
2+ = in between
3+
4+ = relatively common
```

Source: Depression Guideline Panel. *Depression in Primary Care: Detection, Diagnosis, and Treatment*. Quick Reference Guide for Clinicians, Number 5, Rockville, MD. US Department of Health and Human Services, Public Health Service, Agency for Health Care Policy and Research. AHCPR Publication 93-0552. April, 1993.

OUTPATIENT MANAGEMENT
Charting Pearls
Each visit document:
• fetal heart tones and fetal movement
• √ blood pressure, urine dipstick protein
• outstanding lab results
• presentation and fundal height
• estimated gestational age
• date of return visit
• type of uterine incision if previous cesarean section
• discussion regarding postpartum contraception
• discussion of VBAC if previous low transverse C/S
• cervical exam if preterm labor symptoms present
• presence or absence of preterm labor symptoms, bleeding, vaginal discharge or SROM
• presence or absence of symptoms of preeclampsia (PIH)
  • blurred vision
  • scotoma
  • headache
  • rapid weight gain and edema

Routine Prenatal Laboratories

First Visit	Comments
Type and screen	
Rubella	Administer vaccine postpartum
VDRL	Same as RPR
HBsAg	
HIV	
Pap smear	
Cervical cultures for GC and chlamydia	Include Group B strep depending on clinic protocol
Complete blood count	
Hemoglobin electrophoresis	Where indicated
PPD	
Discuss genetic screening	e.g Tay-Sachs, Canavan's, cystic fibrosis, risk for aneuploidy and CVS vs. amniocentesis
16-20 weeks gestation	
Offer MSAFP or "triple screen"	Triple screen = AFP + estriol + free ß-HCG
18-20 weeks gestation	
Ultrasound examination	As indicated
24-28 weeks gestation	
1 hour glucose challenge	See comments on page 57
28-30 weeks	
RhoGAM administration	Must have negative antibody screen prior to RhoGAM
33-37 weeks	
Group B strep culture	If following prenatal screening algorithm
Repeat CBC	
36-40 weeks	
Repeat VDRL	In high-risk patients

OBSTETRICS

NAUSEA AND VOMITING IN PREGNANCY

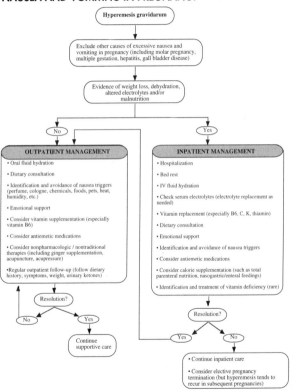

Source: Modified from Erick, M. Hyperemesis gravidarum: a practical management strategy. *OBG Management*, November 2000, 25-35. Reproduced with permission of Dr. Errol Norwitz, Department of Maternal Fetal Medicine, Brigham and Women's Hospital, Boston, MA.

NAUSEA AND VOMITING IN PREGNANCY

Therapy	Route of Administration / Dose	Efficacy	Comments
Anti-emetics			
Metaclopramide (Reglan)	PO (10-30 mg qid) IM/IV (10 mg q 4-6 hr)	Effective	Concern over possible teratogenic effects not well founded in humans, often given with hydroxyzine (Aterax), 25-50 mg q 4-6 hr
Ondansetron (Zofran)	PO (4-8 mg q 4-8 hr) IV (8 mg q 4-8 hr)	Probably effective	A serotonin receptor antagonist, common side effects include mild sedation and headache
Droperidol (Inapsine)	IV/IM (2.5 mg q 3-6 hr IV continuous infusion (1-2.5 mg/h)	Probably effective	No known teratogenicity
Phenothiazines / Antipsychotics			
Promethazine (Phenergan)	PO/PR/IM (12.5-50 mg q 4-6 hr)	Effective	No known teratogenicity, may cause extrapyramidal (Parkinsonian) side effects, hypertension, sedation
Prochlorperazine (Compazine)	PO/IV/IM (5-10 mg q 4-6 hr) PR (25 mg q 12 hr)	Probably effective	No known teratogenicity
Chlorpromazine (Thorazine)	PO/IM (10-50 mg q 6-8 hr)	Probably effective	No known teratogenicity
Antihistamines			
Doxylamine succinate (Unisom)	PO (12.5-25 mg daily)	Probably effective	No known teratogenicity
Doxylamine succinate 10 mg + pyridoxine 10 mg (Bendectin)	PO (1-2 tablets q 6-8 hr)	Effective	Initial concern over teratogenic effects not well founded in humans
Meclizine (Antivert)	PO (25-100 mg daily)	Possibly effective	No known teratogenicity
Chlorpheniramine (Chlor-Trimeton)	PO (8-12 mg daily)	Possibly effective	No known teratogenicity
Diphenhydramine (Dramamine)	PO/IM/IV (50-75 mg q 4-6 hr)	Possibly effective	No known teratogenicity
Trimethobenzamide (Tigan)	PO (250 mg tid/qid) PR/IM (200 mg q 6-8 hr)	Possibly effective	No known teratogenicity

Source: Modified from Erick, M. Hyperemesis gravidarum: a practical management strategy. *OBG Management*, November 2000, 25-35. Reproduced with permission of Dr. Errol Norwitz, Department of Maternal Fetal Medicine, Brigham and Women's Hospital, Boston, MA.

OBSTETRICS

NUTRITION
Weight Gain
- recommendations based on Body Mass Index (BMI) or ideal body weight (IBW)
- prepregnancy values are the only values with documented clinical significance
- adolescents should strive for gains at the upper end of the range
- short women (<157 cm or 62") should aim for the lower end of the range
- obese women should gain at least 6 kg

Prepregnancy Weight	IBW (%)	BMI	Recommended net weight gain
Underweight	< 90	< 19.8	12-18 kg
Acceptable	90-120	19.8-26.0	11-16 kg
Overweight	121-135	26.0-29.0	7-11 kg
Severely overweight	> 135	> 29.0	7 kg

Excessive weight gain	> 1.5 kg/mo
Inadequate weight gain	< 0.25 kg/wk or < 1kg/mo

Caloric Requirements
- 1st and early 2nd trimester   25-30 kcal/kg IBW
- late 2nd and early 3rd   25-35 kcal/kg IBW

Iron Supplementation
- total iron requirement during pregnancy = 1000 mg
  - 30 mg of elemental iron/day recommended during second and third trimesters
    - 150 mg ferrous sulfate or
    - 300 mg ferrous gluconate or
    - 100 mg ferrous fumarate

Folate Supplementation
- routine supplementation is now recommended for all women of reproductive age
  - (0.4 mg/day = amount in most prenatal vitamins)
- history of neural tube defects
  - begin prepregnancy (*MMWR* 40: 513-16, 1991)
  - 4 mg daily

Special Needs
- vitamin D - 10 μg (400 IU) daily for complete vegetarians
- vitamin B12 - 2 μg daily for complete vegetarians
- calcium - 600 mg daily for women < 25 years old with < 600 mg daily by diet

CLINICAL PELVIMETRY

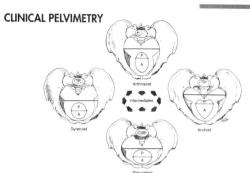

Source: Cunningham FG, MacDonald PC, Gant NF et al. Anatomy of the female reproductive tract. In: *Williams Obstetrics.* 20th ed. Stamford, Conn.: Appleton & Lange, 1997. Reproduced with permission of the publisher.

Classification	Forepelvis	Sidewalls	Sacrum Inclination	Sacrosciatic Notch	Ischial Spines	Arch
Gynecoid	wide	straight	medium	medium	not prominent	wide
Android	narrow	convergent	forward	narrow	prominent	narrow
Anthropoid	narrow	divergent	backward	wide	not prominent	medium
Platypelloid	wide	straight	forward	narrow	not prominent	medium

Pelvic Plane	Diameter	Average Length (cm)
Inlet	True conjugate	11.5
	Obstetric conjugate	11
	Transverse	13.5
	Oblique	12.5
		4.5
Greatest diameter	A-P	12.75
	Transverse	12.5
Mid-plane	A-P	12
	Bispinous	10
	Posterior sagittal	4.5-5
Outlet	Anatomic A-P	9.5
	Obstetric A-P	11.5
	Bituberous	11
	Posterior sagittal	7.5

Source: Bochner C. Anatomic characteristics of the fetal head and maternal pelvis. In: Hacker NF, Moore JG, ed. *Essentials of Obstetrics and Gynecology.* 2nd ed. Philadelphia: Saunders, 1992. Reproduced with permission of the publisher.

OBSTETRICS

INDUCTION OF LABOR

Fast Facts
• overall rate of induction has increased to 184/1000 live births in 1997
• induction indicated for various maternal/fetal conditions
• Bishop score ≥ 6 favorable for success

PGE$_2$ Gel (Prepidil Gel)
• dinoprostone 0.5 mg/3 g gel
• preloaded syringe with 2.5 ml of gel
    • applied with shielded catheter
    • 0.5 mg intracervical dose
    • apply at 6 hour intervals for maximum of 3 doses in 24 hours
• shown to increase Bishop score and rate of successful induction
• no demonstrable decrease in cesarean rate
• wait 6-12 hours after last dose to begin oxytocin
• 1% rate of hyperstimulation

PGE$_2$ Vaginal Insert (Cervidil)
• dinoprostone 10 mg designed for release at 0.3 mg/hr over 3 hours
• vaginal insert placed in posterior fornix
• single application
• carefully monitor uterine activity (5% rate of hyperstimulation)
    • remove for hyperstimulation/fetal distress etc.
• remove after 12 hours then start oxytocin after *at least* 30 minute delay

PGE$_1$ Tablets (Misoprostol)
• same indications and contraindications as for PGE$_2$ use
• 25 mcg to 50 mcg dose
• NOT FDA approved for cervical ripening (See ACOG Committee Opinion 228)
• increased rate of uterine rupture in VBAC candidates
• maintain continuous electronic fetal monitoring
• administer 25 mcg dose every 4-6 hours
• wait 4 hours after the last dose of misoprostol before initiating oxytocin

Foley Catheter
• comparable success to medical methods
• insert sterile speculum and clean cervix with betadine or other antiseptic
• use ring forceps to insert tip of Foley catheter just beyond internal cervical os
• fill balloon over 30-60 minutes with sterile water
• apply gentle traction on the catheter and tape to patient's thigh
• Foley will fall out when cervix has dilated in response to the pressure applied

INDUCTION OF LABOR (CONT.)

Precautions

- document indication, estimated fetal weight (EFW) and presentation (by ultrasound) clearly in chart
- if elective induction, document lung maturity if < 39 weeks
- normal fetal heart rate prior to placement
- monitor fetal heart rate and uterine activity for at least 30 minutes to 2 hours after administration of gel or continuously with misoprostol
- use caution in patients with asthma, glaucoma, or renal, pulmonary and hepatic disease

Bishop Scoring for Cervical Ripening

Factor	0	1	2	3
Cervical Dilation (cm)	closed	1-2	3-4	5+
Cervical Effacement (%)	0-30	40-50	60-70	80+
Fetal Station	-3	-2	-1	+1, +2
Cervical Consistency	firm	medium	soft	•
Cervical Position	posterior	mid	anterior	•

Add 1 point for: preeclampsia, each prior vaginal delivery
Deduct 1 point for: postdates, nulliparity, preterm or prolonged PROM

Predictive value for success

Score
0-4	45-50% failure
5-9	10% failure
10-13	0% failure

OBSTETRICS

FETAL LUNG MATURITY

Fetal maturity may be assumed and amniocentesis need not be performed if **one** of the
following is met:

1. Fetal heart tones have been documented for 20 weeks by non-electric fetoscope or for 30
   weeks by Doppler.
2. It has been 36 weeks since a positive serum or urine human chorionic gonadotropin (hCG)
   pregnancy test was performed by a reliable laboratory.
3. An ultrasound measurement of the crown-rump length, obtained at 6-11 weeks, supports a
   gestational age of > 39 weeks.
4. An ultrasound, obtained at 12-20 weeks, confirms the gestational age of >39 weeks
   determined by clinical history and physical exam.

From Fetal Maturity Assessment Prior to Elective Repeat Cesarean Birth. ACOG Committee Opinion #98, September 1991.

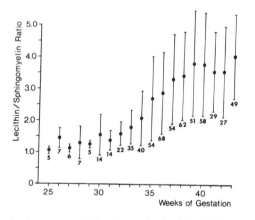

Source: Donald IR, Freeman RK, Goebelsmann U, et al. Clinical experience with the amniotic fluid lecithin-sphingomyelin ratio. I. Antenatal
prediction of pulmonary maturity. *Am J Obstet Gynecol* 1973;115(4):547-52. Reproduced with permission of the publisher, Mosby-Year
Book: St. Louis.

FETAL LUNG MATURITY (CONT.)

Test	Technique	Threshold	Typical Predictive Value		Notes
			Mature	Immature	
Lecithin/sphingomyelin ratio	Thin-layer chromatography	2.0-3.5	95-100	33-50	Many variations in technique; laboratory variation significant
Phosphatidylglycerol	Thin-layer chromatography	"Present" (usually means >3% of total phospholipid)	95-100	23-53	Not affected by blood, meconium; vaginal pool samples satisfactory
	Antisera	0.5=low positive 2.0=high positive	95-100	23-53	Not affected by blood, meconium; vaginal pool samples satisfactory
Foam stability index	Ethanol added to amniotic fluid, solution shaken, presence of stable bubbles at meniscus noted	47 or 48	95	51	Affected by blood, meconium, vaginal pool debris, silicone-coated test tubes
Fluorescence polarization	Fluorescence polarization	55 mg/g of albumin	96-100	47,61	Minimal intraassay and interassay variability; simple testing procedure
Optical density (OD) at 650 nm	Spectrophotometric reading	OD 0.15	98	13	Simple technique
Lamellar body counts	Counts using commercial hematology counter	30,000-40,000 (still investigational)	97-98	29-35	Promising technique

Source: American College of Obstetricians and Gynecologists: *Assessment of Fetal Lung Maturity.* Educational Bulletin 230. ACOG, Washington, DC © 1996. Reproduced with permission of the publisher.

OBSTETRICS

CHROMOSOMAL ABNORMALITIES AT AMNIOCENTESIS

Maternal Age	SINGLETON GESTATION		TWIN GESTATION	
	Trisomy 21	All Abnormalities	Trisomy 21	All Abnormalities
25	1/885	1/1533	1/481	1/833
26	1/826	1/1202	1/447	1/650
27	1/769	1/943	1/415	1/509
28	1/719	1/740	1/387	1/398
29	1/680	1/580	1/364	1/310
30	1/641	1/455	1/342	1/243
31	1/610	1/357	1/324	1/190
32	1/481	1/280	1/256	1/149
33	1/389	1/219	1/206	1/116
34	1/303	1/172	1/160	1/91
35	1/237	1/135	1/125	1/71
36	1/185	1/106	1/98	1/56
37	1/145	1/83	1/77	1/44
38	1/113	1/65	1/60	1/35
39	1/89	1/51	1/47	1/27
40	1/69	1/40	1/37	1/21
41	1/55	1/31	1/29	1/17
42	1/43	1/25	1/23	1/13
43	1/33	1/19	1/18	1/10
44	1/26	1/15	1/14	1/8
45	1/21	1/12	1/11	1/6

Source: Meyers C, Adam R, Dungan J, Prenger V. Aneuploidy in twin gestations: When is maternal age advanced? *Obstet Gynecol.* 1997;89:248-251. Reproduced with permission from the American College of Obstetricians and Gynecologists.

ANEUPLOID RISK OF MAJOR ANOMALIES

Structural Defect	Population Incidence	Aneuploidy Risk	Most Common Aneuploidy
Cystic hygroma	1/120 EU - 1/6,000 B	60-70%	45X (80%); 21, 18, 13, XXY
Hydrops	1/1,500-4,000 B	30-80%*	13, 21, 18, 45X
Hydrocephalus	3-8/10,000 LB	3-8%	13, 18, triploidy
Hydranencephaly	2/1,000 IA	Minimal	
Holoprosencephaly	1/16,000 LB	40-60%	13, 18, 18p-
Cardiac defects	7-9/1,000 LB	5-30%	21, 18, 13, 22, 8, 9
Complete arterioventricular canal		40-70%	21
Diaphragmatic hernia	1/3,500-4,000 LB	20-25%	13, 18, 21, 45X
Omphalocele	1/5,800 LB	30-40%	13, 18
Gastroschisis	1/10,000-15,000 LB	Minimal	
Duodenal atresia	1/10,000 LB	20-30%	21
Bowel obstruction	1/2,500-5,000 LB	Minimal	
Bladder outlet obstruction	1-2/1,000 LB	20-25%	13, 18
Prune belly syndrome	1/35,000-50,000 LB	Low	18, 13, 45X
Facial cleft	1/700 LB	1%	13, 18, deletions
Limb reduction	4-6/10,000 LB	8%	18
Club foot	1.2/1,000 LB	6%	18, 13, 4p-, 18q-
Single umbilical artery	1%	Minimal	

Abbreviations: EU, early ultrasound; B, birth; LB, livebirth; IA, infant autopsy

*30% if diagnosed ≥ 24 weeks; 80% if diagnosed ″ ≤ 17 weeks

Data from Shipp TD, Benacerraf BR. The significance of prenatally identified isolated clubfoot: is amniocentesis indicated? *Am J Obstet Gynecol.* 1998;178:600-602; and Nyberg DA, Crane JP. Chromosomal abnormalities. In: Nyberg DA, Mahony BS, Pretorius DH. *Diagnostic Ultrasound of Fetal Anomalies: text and atlas.* Chicago: Year Book Medical, 1990:676-724.

Source: American College of Obstetricians and Gynecologists. *Prenatal Diagnosis of Fetal Chromosomal Abnormalities.* ACOG Practice Bulletin Number 27, May 2001. Reproduced with permission of the American College of Obstetricians and Gynecologists.

OBSTETRICS

TRIPLE MARKER SCREENING
Neural Tube Defects
• occur in 1/1,500 live births in California
• anencephaly and spina bifida account for 95% of neural tube defects
• 95% of infants with NTD's are born into families with no previous history
• folic acid dietary supplementation reduces incidence of neural tube defects

Abdominal Wall Defects
• two types: omphalocele and gastroschisis
• omphalocele is a protrusion into the umbilical cord while gastroschisis occurs to the right of the cord
• rate of abdominal wall defects is 1/2,500 live births in California

Chromosomal Abnormalities
• risk increases with maternal age
• trisomy 21 occurs in 1/700 California live births, trisomy 18 in 1/6,500 live births in California
• 70% of trisomy 18 fetuses miscarry before birth, mean survival is 48 days with 5-10% surviving 1 year
• any couple with a family history of any chromosomal abnormality should be referred for genetic counseling

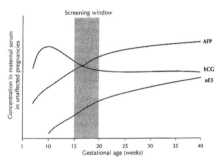

AFP	hCG	uE3	Condition
▼	▲	▲	Down syndrome
▲	not used	not used	Open neural tube defects Abdominal wall defects
▼	▼	▼	Trisomy 18

Source: The California Expanded AFP Screening Program Prenatal Care Provider Handbook.
California Department of Health Services, Genetic Disease Branch

MATERNAL SERUM EXPANDED AFP SCREENING

Maternal Age at EDD (years)	Observed Screen Positive Rates (%)[+]	Expected Detection Rates (%) [*]
20	2.3	40
21	1.8	41
22	1.8	41
23	2.1	42
24	2.2	43
25	2.2	44
26	2.3	45
27	2.3	46
28	2.5	47
29	2.9	50
30	2.9	52
31	3.5	55
32	4.6	58
33	5.6	62
34	6.9	66
35	9.3	71
36	11.3	75
37	15.1	79
38	18.9	83
39	21.7	87
40	25.9	90
41	31.8	92
42	35.4	95
43	41.1	96
44	50.0	99
45	52.7	99
46	77.4	99
<35	3.0	50
35	17.8	85
All ages	4.1	66

• combining MSAFP, hCG and unconjugated estriol forms the basis of the "triple screen" test

+ January-June 1996
* If all screen-positive women accept amniocentesis

Source: The California Expanded AFP Screening Program Prenatal Care Provider Handbook. California Department of Health Services, Genetic Disease Branch

OBSTETRICS

LABOR AND DELIVERY
Labor-Normal
- ideally each patient should be evaluated at least q 2 hr (with or without an exam)
- labor is a physiologic not pathologic process
- see the Friedman curve as detailed below:

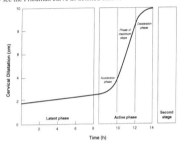

Source: Friedman EA. *Labor: Evaluation and Management*, 2nd edition. East Norwalk CT: Appleton-Century-Crofts, 1978. Reproduced with the permission of the publisher.

Avoid unnecessary examinations and remember the following (Courtesy of S. Joel-Cohen)

5 C's	5 P's
Clean (first)	Presentation
Catheterize (or empty bladder, second)	Position
Cervix (effacement, dilation...)	Place (station)
Caput (is it head or caput?)	Pelvis (clinical pelvimetry)
Cord (are there cord pulsations beyond membranes?)	Puncture (SROM or need for amniotomy)

Labor-Dysfunctional

Pattern	Nulligravida	Multiparous	Therapeutic Interventions
Prolonged Latent Phase	> 20 hours	> 14 hours	Rest, oxytocin
Protraction Disorder			
Dilation	< 1.2 cm/hr	< 1.5 cm/hr	AROM, oxytocin
Descent	< 1cm/hr	< 2 cm/hr	Oxytocin
Arrest Disorder *			
Dilation	> 2 hours	> 2 hours	AROM, oxytocin, cesarean section
Descent	> 2 hours	> 1 hour	Forceps, vacuum, cesarean section
	> 3 hours with epidural	> 2 hours with epidural	

* With documented adequate uterine contractions: >200 Montevideo units/10 minutes for 2 hours

Source: American College of Obstetricians and Gynecologists: *Dystocia*. Technical Bulletin 137. ACOG, Washington, DC © 1989. Reproduced with the permission of the publisher. and American College of Obstetricians and Gynecologists: *Operative Vaginal Delivery*. ACOG Practice Bulletin #17, June 2000. ACOG, Washington, DC © 2000.

OBSTETRICS

SHOULDER DYSTOCIA

Definition:
Failure of the shoulders to deliver spontaneously with usual methods, secondary to impaction of the anterior shoulder behind the symphysis pubis

Incidence:
0.5 - 2.9% of all deliveries

Risk Factors:
Maternal obesity, diabetes, history of macrosomic infant, current macrosomia

Risk of Shoulder Dystocia (%) as a Function of Birthweight

Reference	2500-2999 g	3000-3499 g	3500-3999 g	4000-4499 g	4500-5000 g	>5000 g
Acker DB et al. *Obstet Gynecol* 1985;66(6):762-8.	0.2	0.6	2.3	10.3	23.9	
Spellacy WN et al. *Obstet Gynecol* 1985;66(2):158-61.	0.3		N/A		7.3	14.6
Benedetti TJ et al. *Obstet Gynecol* 198=78;52(5):526-9.	1.5		3.0			

- 2/3 occur with birthweight < 4000 g
- diabetic pregnancies are at higher risk

Warning Signs: (ANTICIPATION IS KEY)
• prolonged 2nd stage of labor • recoil of head on perineum (turtle sign) • lack of spontaneous restitution

Treatment:
1) McRobert's Maneuver - dorsiflexion on hips against abdomen
2) Cut generous episiotomy
3) Suprapubic pressure (**NOT** fundal pressure)
4) Constant moderate **DOWNWARD** traction to count of 30
5) Rubin's Screw Maneuver (rotate face towards floor)
6) Attempt Wood's Screw with extraction of posterior arm (may fracture humerus)
7) Zavenelli Maneuver - cephalic replacement/abdominal rescue

HELPER Alogorithm (Courtesy of Dr. Khoa Lai)
H elp
E pisiotomy
L eg elevated (McRobert's)
P ressure (suprapubic)
E nter vagina and attempt rotation (Wood's screw)
R each for fetal arm

OBSTETRICS

OPERATIVE VAGINAL DELIVERY

Criteria for Types of Forceps Delivery

Outlet forceps

1. Scalp is visible at the introitus without separating the labia
2. Fetal skull has reached the pelvic floor.
3. Sagittal suture is in an anteroposterior diameter or right or left occiput anterior or posterior position.
4. Rotation does not exceed 45°.

Low forceps

Leading point of fetal skull is at station ≥ +2cm, and not on the pelvic floor.
Rotation is 45° or less (left or right occiput anterior to occiput anterior, or left or right occiput posterior to occiput posterior.
Rotation is greater than 45°.

Mid forceps

Station above + 2cm but head is engaged.

High forceps

Not included in classification.

Source: American College of Obstetricians and Gynecologists: *Operative Vaginal Delivery*. ACOG Practice Bulletin #17, June 2000. ACOG, Washington, DC © 2000.

Tips from Dr. Shirley Tom
• have clear indication for forceps (fetal distress, prolonged 2nd stage, etc.)
• have good anesthesia
• empty the bladder
• know fetal position precisely (feel for fetal ear helix if caput present)

Indications for Operative Vaginal Delivery

No indication for operative vaginal delivery is absolute. The following indications apply when the head is engaged and the cervix fully dilated.

Prolonged second stage

Nulliparous women	Lack of continuing progress for 3 hours with regional anestheia, or 2 hours without regional anesthesia
Multiparous women	Lack of continuing progress for 2 hours with regional anesthesia, or 1 hour without regional anesthesia

Suspicion of immediate or potential fetal compromise

Shortening of the second stage for maternal benefit

Source: American College of Obstetricians and Gynecologists: *Operative Vaginal Delivery*. ACOG Practice Bulletin #17, June 2000. ACOG, Washington, DC © 2000. Reproduced with permission.

TYPES OF FORCEPS

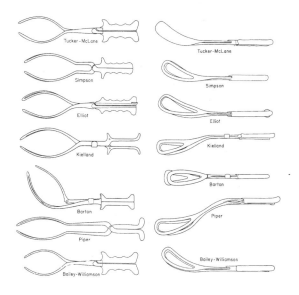

Tucker-McLane

Tucker-McLane

Simpson

Simpson

Elliot

Elliot

Kielland

Kielland

Barton

Barton

Piper

Piper

Bailey-Williamson

Bailey-Williamson

From Zuspan FP, Quilligan EJ. Forceps. In: *Douglas-Stromme Operative Obstetrics* 5th ed. Norwalk, Conn.: Appleton & Lange, 1988. Reproduced with the permission of the publisher.

OBSTETRICS

VACUUM EXTRACTION

Fast Facts
- use same indications as forceps, but ease of application has clouded judgment of some physicians
- all cups are approximately 6 cm in diameter
- can result in fetal injuries similar to forceps, higher incidence of scalp injuries
  - cephalohematoma in 14-16% of vacuum deliveries (vs. 2% with forceps)
  - subgaleal hematoma in 26-45/1,000 vacuum deliveries
  - retinal hemorrhages in 38% (vs. 17% with forceps)

Application and Delivery
- know the fetal position exactly
- check manufacturer's recommendations
- position cup symmetrically over sagittal suture 3 cm anterior to posterior fontanelle: "flexion point"
- apply low suction (100 mm Hg) increase pressure to 500 mm Hg and pull along pelvic curve
- check that no vaginal or cervical tissue is trapped by cup
- descent of the head must occur with each pull
- delivery should be accomplished with 3-5 pulls
- maximum of 3 "pop-offs"
- head should be completely delivered within 15 minutes of first application
- do not use for rotation
- avoid rocking movements or excessive torque

Relative Contraindications
- prematurity (<37 weeks)
- suspected macrosomia
- suspected fetal coagulation disorder
- fetal scalp sampling
- non-vertex presentation

Delivery Method	Neonatal Death	Intracranial Hemorrhage	Other*
Spontaneous vaginal delivery	1/5,000	1/1,900	1/216
Cesarean delivery during labor	1/1,250	1/952	1/71
Cesarean delivery after vacuum/forceps	N/R	1/333	1/38
Cesarean delivery with no labor	1/1,250	1/2,040	1/105
Vacuum alone	1/3,333	1/860	1/122
Forceps alone	1/2,000	1/664	1/76
Vacuum and forceps	1/1,666	1/280	1/58

Abbreviation: N/R indicates not reported

*Facial nerve/brachial plexus injury, convulsions, central nervous system depression, mechanical ventilation

Data from Towner D, Castro MA, Eby-Wilkens E, Gilbert WM. Effect of mode of delivery in nulliparous women on neonatal intracranial brain injury. *N Engl J Med* 1999; 341:1709-1714.

Source: American College of Obstetricians and Gynecologists: *Operative Vaginal Delivery*. ACOG Practice Bulletin #17, June 2000. ACOG, Washington, DC © 2000.

CESAREAN SECTION

Fast Facts
- origin of term remains mysterious
  - method of delivery of Julius Caesar (certainly a myth)
  - *lex cesarea* - Roman law requiring removal of fetus from dead mother
  - derived from Latin verb *caedere* "to cut"

- historical high points
  - 1896 E. Pouro introduces cesarean hysterectomy (maternal mortality 15%)
  - 1907 F. Frank extraperitoneal cesarean section
  - 1912 B. Kronig bladder displacement with vertical uterine incision
  - 1926 J. Kerr transverse uterine incision (downward curving)
  - 1931 L. Phaneuf modern style low transverse incision

- maternal mortality low (less than 1/5000)
- primary cesarean section rates higher than 25% in some centers

Indications
- be precise, be specific
- write a detailed pre-operative note

Fetal

fetal distress (specify abnormality-recurrent late decels, bradycardia, etc.)
fetal intolerance of labor
inability to document fetal well-being
malpresentation (breech, transverse lie)
twins (non-vertex first twin, possibly for non-vertex 2nd twin)
maternal HSV infection
fetal congenital anomalies

Maternal-fetal

labor abnormalities
- active phase arrest
- arrest of descent
- failed induction
- inefficient uterine contractility unresponsive to therapy

placental abruption (certain cases)
placenta previa
pelvic malformation (absolute pelvic disproportion)
estimated fetal weight > 4500g (controversial)

Maternal

obstructive benign/malignant tumors
severe vulvar condylomata
cervical carcinoma
abdominal cerclage
prior vaginal colporrhaphy
vaginal delivery contraindicated (medical indications)

OBSTETRICS

CESAREAN SECTION
Uterine Incision
- most common: low transverse (A) or Kerr (D)
- low vertical (B)
  - premature fetus with malpresentation or poorly developed lower segment
  - usually extends into active segment
- classical (C)
  - rarely used
  - impacted transverse lie, cervical carcinoma

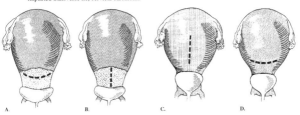

Source: Scott JR. Cesarean delivery. In: Scott JR, DiSaia PD, Hammond CB, Spellacy WN, ed. *Danforth's Obstetrics and Gynecology.* 7th ed. Philadelphia: Lippincott, 1994. Reproduced with the permission of the publisher.

Druzin Splint Maneuver
- malpresentations in premature fetus often associated with difficult delivery
- choose correct uterine incision
- Druzin splint technique as detailed below to allow atraumatic delivery
  - breech or transverse lie
  - intact membranes helpful

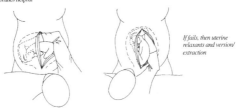

If fails, then uterine relaxants and version/extraction

Source: Druzin ML. Atraumatic delivery in cases of malpresentation of the very low birth weight fetus at cesarean section: the splint technique. *Am J Obstet Gynecol* 1986;154(4):941-2. Reproduced with the permission of the publisher, Mosby-Year Book: St. Louis.

36

VAGINAL BIRTH AFTER CESAREAN (VBAC)
Candidates
• Trial of Labor (TOL) recommended in most cases after previous low transverse incision
• internal fetal monitoring strongly suggested
• use of pitocin not contraindicated
• remember: *a scarred uterus is not a normal uterus*

Complications and Success Rate
• uterine rupture is rare (<1%) with one previous low transverse incision
• risk of rupture increases to ~2% with 2 previous C/S
    • uterine rupture most commonly associated with variable decels and/or bradycardia
• use of an intrauterine pressure catheter (IUPC) does not predict rupture but can be useful in
    documenting adequate contractions in arrest disorders
• success rates vary with indications of previous section (9)
    • non-recurrent indications (breech): 85% success
    • previous arrest disorder (CPD): 67%

Recommendations from ACOG
The following recommendations are based on good and consistent scientific evidence (Level A):
• Most women with one previous cesarean delivery with a low transverse incision are candidates for
    VBAC and should be counseled about VBAC and offered a trial of labor.
• Epidural anesthesia may be used for VBAC.
• A previous uterine incision extending into the fundus is a contraindication for VBAC.

The following recommendations are based on limited or inconsistent scientific evidence (Level B):
• Women with two previous low-transverse cesarean deliveries and no contraindications who wish to
    attempt VBAC may be allowed a trial of labor. They should be advised that the risk of
    uterine rupture increases as the number of cesarean deliveries increases.
• Use of oxytocin or prostaglandin gel for VBAC requires close patient monitoring.
• Women with a vertical incision within the lower uterine segment that does not extend into the
    fundus are candidates for VBAC.

The following recommendations are based primarily on consensus and expert opinion (Level C):
• Because uterine rupture may be catastrophic, VBAC should be attempted in institutions equipped
    to respond to emergencies with physicians immediately available to provide emergency care.
• After thorough counseling that weighs the individual benefits and risks of VBAC, the ultimate
    decision to attempt this procedure or undergo a repeat cesarean delivery should be made by
    the patient and her physician.

Sources: *Vaginal Birth After Previous Cesarean Delivery.* ACOG Committee Opinion Number 238, July 2000. (Replaces Committee Opinion No. 168, February 1996) and ACOG Practice Bulletin Number 5, July 1999 *Vaginal Birth After Previous Cesarean Delivery.*

Maurice L. Druzin says, "Do it My Way" (with apologies to Sinatra)
• Appropriate candidates
• Informed consent x 2
• Honest appraisal of risk

• Schedule elective repeat C/S at 41 weeks (if not in spontaneous labor)
• Induction, use mechanical methods
• Augmentation with oxytocin is acceptable
• 24/7 coverage (Obstetrics, Anesthesia, operating room)

OBSTETRICS

POST PARTUM HEMORRHAGE

Definition
≥500 cc blood loss in first 24 hours after delivery

Etiology and Risk Factors

1. Atony
- grand multiparity
- uterine overdistention
- prolonged labor with pitocin augmentation
- chorioamnionitis
- general anesthesia
- $MgSO_4$ therapy for seizure prophylaxis
- rapid labor

2. Retained placental tissue
- usually delayed postpartum hemorrhage
- placenta accreta (especially multiple prior cesareans)
- preterm delivery
- succenturiate lobe
- cord avulsion

3. Genital tract laceration
- precipitous labor and delivery
- improper episiotomy repair
- operative vaginal delivery

4. Uterine inversion - Don't pull on that cord!

Treatment

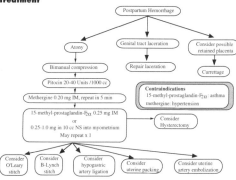

UTERINE ARTERY LIGATION
Inserting the Suture

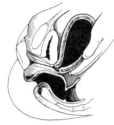

Figure 1. Grasp and elevate the uterus with the left hand and tilt it to expose the vessels.

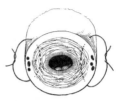

Figure 2. A coronal view of lower uterine segment is shown. Insert the suture into the substance of the cervix without entering the uterine cavity and medial to the blood vessels

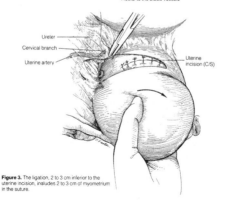

Ureter

Cervical branch

Uterine artery

Uterine incision (C/S)

Figure 3. The ligation, 2 to 3 cm inferior to the uterine incision, inaludes 2 to 3 cm of myometrium in the suture.

Source: O'Leary JA. Stop OB hemorrhage with uterine artery ligation. *Cont Ob/Gyn* Special Issue: Update on Surgery 1986. Reproduced with the permission of the publisher, Medical Economics Publishing: Montvale, N.J.

OBSTETRICS

B-LYNCH SUTURE FOR POSTPARTUM HEMORRHAGE

FIGURE 1
Anterior 3/4 view

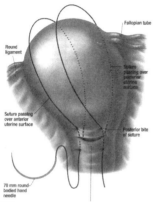
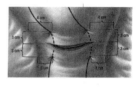

FIGURE 2
Posterior 3/4 view

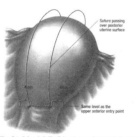

Source: Chez RA, B-Lynch C. The B-Lynch suture for control of massive postpartum hemorrhage. *Cont Ob/Gyn* 1998; August: 93-98. Reproduced with permission of Mr. Philip Wilson, F.M.A.A., R.M.I.P.

OBSTETRICS

LOWER UTERINE SEGMENT PACKING

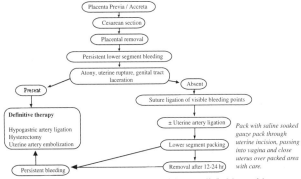

Pack with saline soaked gauze pack through uterine incision, passing into vagina and close uterus over packed area with care.

Source: Modified from Druzin ML. Packing of lower uterine segment for control of postcesarean bleeding in instances of placenta previa. *Surg Gynecol Obstet* 1989;169(6):543-5. Reproduced with the permission of *Surgery, Gynecology & Obstetrics*, now known as the *Journal of the American College of Surgeons.*

UTERINE INVERSION
Fast Facts
• 1/25,000 deliveries
• more common multips
• often iatrogenic

Presentation
• placenta appears at introitus with mass attached
• shock with bradycardia 2° to vagal response
• excessive hemorrhage

Treatment
• treat for shock and blood loss
• call for assistance (especially anesthesia)
• administer uterine relaxants
    • terbutaline 0.25 mg IV (may repeat x 1)
    • nitroglycerine 100-250 µg IV up to total of 1000 µg (watch BP)
• replace uterus
    • "last out, first in"
    • pressure applied around, NOT at, leading point
    • may require general anesthesia (Halothane)
    • do not remove placenta if firmly attached until uterus replaced
• exploratory laparotomy with replacement if all else fails

OBSTETRICS

EMERGENCY CERCLAGE

Fast Facts
• method to perform cerclage in face of prolapsed membranes
• heroic measure

Inclusion Criteria
• intact membranes
• no evidence of chorioamnionitis
• advanced dilation
• history compatible with incompetent cervix (not preterm labor)
• no gross fetal anomalies
• extreme prematurity

Preparation
• informed consent
• general or regional anesthesia
• perineal and vaginal prep

Technique
• steep Trendelenburg position
• insert Foley into bladder
• backfill bladder with 1/2 NS in 250 cc increments
• membranes usually recede after 800-1000 cc
• place cerclage (McDonald or Shirodkar)

Post-Operative Care
• empty bladder
• antibiotics
• prophylactic tocolytics

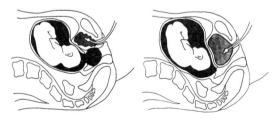

Source: Scheerer LJ, Lam F, Bartolucci L, et al. A new technique for reduction of prolapsed fetal membranes for emergency cervical cerclage. *Obstet Gynecol*, 1989; 74(3): 408-10. Reproduced with the permission of the American College of Obstetricians and Gynecologists.

OBSTETRICS

AMNIOINFUSION

Fast Facts
- attempt to prevent problems in labor associated with oligohydramnios
- reduction in cesarean section rate for fetal distress by reducing variable decelerations

Candidates for Amnioinfusion
- preterm PROM with ultrasound-demonstrated oligohydramnios
- term labor with recurrent variable decels and decreased amniotic fluid
- cephalic presentation
- previous cesarean section or previous myomectomy not an absolute contraindication
- chorioamnionitis is a relative contraindication

Technique
- document fetal presentation and oligohydramnios by ultrasound
- place fetal scalp electrode and intrauterine pressure catheter (preferably double lumen catheter)
- initial bolus of 250-500 cc of normal saline (warmed) with maintenance infusion (3 cc/min)
- rebolus as needed
- measure intrauterine pressure every 30 minutes or continuously (second IUPC or double lumen)

	Beneficial	Uncertain	No Benefit
Therapeutic			
Repetitive variable decelerations	•		
Chorioamnionitis		•	
Severe oligohydramnios	•		
Failed version		•	
Prophylaxis			
Preterm premature rupture of membranes		•	
Term oligohydramnios			•
Meconium			•

Source: Spong CY. Amnioinfusion: indications and controversies. *Cont Ob/Gyn* August 1997; 138-159. Reproduced with permission of Medical Economics Publishing.

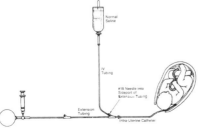

Source: Miyazaki FS, Nevarez F. Saline amnioinfusion for relief of repetitive variable decelerations: a prospective randomized study. *Am J Obstet Gynecol* 1985;153(3):301-6. Reproduced with the permission of the publisher, Mosby-Year Book: St. Louis.

OBSTETRICS

UMBILICAL CORD GAS VALUES

Value	Yeomans (1985)[*] (n=146)	Ramin (1989)[*] (n=1,292)	Riley (1993)[§] (n=3,522)
Arterial blood in term newborns (Mean ± one standard deviation)			
pH	7.28 ± 0.05	7.28 ± 0.07	7.27 ± 0.069
PCO_2 (mm Hg)	49.2 ± 8.4	49.9 ± 14.2	50.3 ± 11.1
HCO_3^- (meq/l)	22.3 ± 2.5	23.1 ± 2.8	22.0 ± 3.6
Base excess (meq/l)	---- [‡]	- 3.6 ± 2.8	- 2.7 ± 2.8
Venous blood in term newborns (Mean ± one standard deviation)			
pH	7.35 ± 0.05	----	7.34 ± 0.063
PCO_2 (mm Hg)	38.2 ± 5.6	----	40.7 ± 7.9
HCO_3^- (meq/l)	20.4 ± 4.1	----	21.4 ± 2.5
Base excess (meq/l)	----	----	- 2.4 ± 2.0

* Data are from infants of selected patients with uncomplicated vaginal deliveries.
§ Data are from infants of unselected patients with vaginal deliveries.
‡ Data were not obtained.

Ramin SM, Gilstrap LC III, Leveno KJ, Burris J, Little BB. Umbilical artery acid-base status in the preterm infant. *Obstet Gynecol* 1989;74:256-258.
Riley RJ, Johnson JWC. Collecting and analyzing cord blood gases. *Clin Obstet Gynecol* 1993;36:13-23.
Yeomans ER, Hauth JC, Gilstrap LC III, Strickland DM. Umbilical cord pH, PCO_2 and bicarbonate following uncomplicated term deliveries. *Am J Obstet Gynecol* 1985;151:798-800.

Value	Ramin (1989)[*] (n=77)	Dickinson (1992)[§] (n=949)	Riley (1993)[§] (n=1,1015)
Arterial blood in preterm newborns (Mean ± one standard deviation)			
pH	7.29 ± 0.07	7.27 ± 0.07	7.28 ± 0.089
PCO_2 (mm Hg)	49.2 ± 9.0	51.6 ± 9.4	50.2 ± 12.3
HCO_3^- (meq/l)	23.0 ± 3.5	23.9 ± 2.1	22.4 ± 3.5
Base excess (meq/l)	-3.3 ± 2.4	- 3.0 ± 2.5	- 2.7 ± 3.0

* Data are from infants of selected patients with uncomplicated vaginal deliveries.
§ Data are from infants of unselected patients with vaginal deliveries.

Dickinson JE, Eriksen NL, Meyer BA, Parisi VM. The effect of preterm birth on umbilical cord blood gases. *Obstet Gynecol* 1992;79:575-578.
Ramin SM, Gilstrap LC III, Leveno KJ, Burris J, Little BB. Umbilical artery acid-base status in the preterm infant. *Obstet Gynecol* 1989;74:256-258.
Riley RJ, Johnson JWC. Collecting and analyzing cord blood gases. *Clin Obstet Gynecol* 1993;36:13-23.

Source: American College of Obstetricians and Gynecologists: *Umbilical Artery Blood Acid-Base Analysis.* ACOG Technical Bulletin #216, November 1995. ACOG, Washington, DC © 2000.

GROUP B STREPTOCOCCUS

Fast Facts

• leading cause of life-threatening perinatal infections in U.S.
• 15-30% of women are asymptomatic carriers
• 7,600 (1.8/1,000 live births) proven neonatal infections per year in U.S.
• early onset infection (80% within 6 hours of delivery) - 6% neonatal mortality
• attack rate increases up to 40/1,000 in cases with multiple risk factors
• two accepted risk reduction strategies as described by the CDC (*MMWR* 45: RR-7, May, 1996)

Prenatal Screening Algorithm

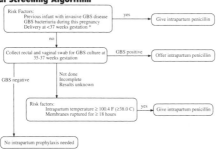

Risk Factor Algorithm

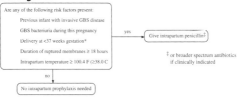

* If membranes ruptured at < 37 weeks gestation, and the mother has not begun labor, collect GBS culture and either
a) administer antibiotics until cultures are completed and the results are negative or b) begin antibiotics only when positive cultures are available.

Choice of Antibiotic Therapy

Recommended: Penicillin G 5 mU IV load, then 2.5 mU IV q 4 hr until delivery
Alternative: Ampicillin 2 g IV load, then 1 g IV q 4 hr until delivery
PCN allergic: Clindamycin 900 mg IV q 8 hr until delivery or Erythromycin 500 mg IV q 6 hr until delivery

OBSTETRICS

INTRA-AMNIOTIC INFECTION

Definition
A bacterial infection of the chorion, amnion and amniotic fluid often diagnosed during a prolonged labor.

Diagnosis
Maternal temperature ≥ 100.7˚F with no other obvious source and one of the following additional findings:
• fetal tachycardia
• maternal tachycardia
• abdominal tenderness
• foul-smelling amniotic fluid
• leukocytosis
• positive amniotic fluid culture

Risk Factors
• Prolonged ruptured of membranes
• Multiple vaginal exams in labor and internal monitoring

Antibiotics
Mezlocillin 4 g IV q 4-6 hr or piperacillin 3-4 g IV q 4 hr
Ticarcillin/clavulanic acid 3.1 g IV q 6 hr
Ampicillin/sulbactam 3 g IV q 4-6 hr
Ampicillin 2 g IV q 6 hr **and** gentamicin 1.5 mg/kg load then 1.0 mg/kg q 8 hr
(if delivery by cesarean section **add** clindamycin 900 mg IV q 6 hr)

Comments
• continue antibiotics for 24-48 hr afebrile following delivery
• chorioamnionitis is **not** an indication for cesarean delivery
• fetal outcome is improved by maternal antibiotic therapy and ↓ temperature
• always consider other sources of maternal fever (pyelonephritis, pneumonia, appendicitis)
• watch for postpartum hemorrhage and dystocia secondary to inadequate uterine action
• chorioamnionitis may represent a risk factor for cerebal palsy

FEBRILE MORBIDITY AND ENDOMYOMETRITIS

Definition

Two temperature elevations to $\geq 38^\circ$ C (100.4° F) (outside the 1st 24 hr after delivery)

    or

A temperature of $\geq 38.7^\circ$ C (101.5° F) at any time

Etiology

Seven W's of febrile morbidity
- **W**omb (endomyometritis)
- **W**ind (atelectesis, pneumonia)
- **W**ater (urinary tract infection or pyelonephritis)
- **W**alk (deep vein thrombosis or pulmonary embolism)
- **W**ound (wound infection, episiotomy infection)
- **W**eaning (breast engorgement, mastitis, breast abscess)
- **W**onder (drug fever - wonder drugs)

Evaluation

Physical examination including pelvic exam to rule out hematoma or retained membranes
CBC with differential, urinalysis, urine and blood cultures as indicated
Valve of endometrial cultures unclear (optional)
Chest X-ray, ultrasound as indicated

Treatment

After diagnosis is made of endomyometritis by PELVIC exam...
Cefotetan 1-2 g IV q 12 hr
Mezlocillin 4 g IV q 4-6 hr or piperacillin 3-4 g IV q 4 hr
Ticarcillin/clavulanate 3.1 g IV q 6 hr
Ampicillin/sulbactam 3 g IV q 4-6 hr
Gentamicin 1.5 mg/kg load then 1.0 mg/kg q 8 hr and clindamycin 900 mg IV q 6 hr
(plus ampicillin 2 g IV q 6 hr as needed to cover enterococcus)

Comments

- continue IV antibiotics until 24-48 hours afebrile and improved physical exam
- oral antibiotics following IV antibiotics have not been shown to be of proven value
- if unresponsive following 48-72 hours of IV antibiotics reexamine the patient
  - consider pelvic abscess
  - consider septic pelvic thrombophlebitis
  - consider drug fever

OBSTETRICS

MASTITIS AND BREAST ABSCESS

Fast Facts
- affects 2-3% of nursing mothers
- most frequently seen as a nonepidemic mammary cellulitis
- usually *Staphylococcus aureus*
- other pathogens: β-hemolytic streptococci, *H. influenzae*, *H. parainfluenzae*, *Escherichia coli*, *Klebsiella pneumoniae*
- must distinguish between simple engorgement and infectious process
- outpatient antibiotic therapy usually successful but consider IV antibiotics if unresponsive or patient compliance/tolerance uncertain or patient appears septic

Evaluation

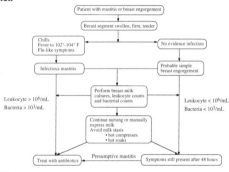

Treatment
- penicillin 250 mg PO qid x 1 week **OR**
- dicloxacillin 250 - 500 mg PO qid x 1 week if suspect penicillin-resistant staphylococci **OR**
- erythromycin 250 mg PO qid x 1 week in penicillin-allergic patient
- breast abscess can form even on antibiotics, surgical drainage necessary

Prevention
- avoid cracked or fissured nipples
  - use plain water to clean nipple area (NOT soap or alcohol)
  - increase duration of nursing gradually to avoid soreness
  - use breast shield or topical cream to help healing of cracked nipples
  - place finger in corner of baby's mouth during feeding to break sucking force
- treat recurrent mastitis promptly but continue breastfeeding

Source: Adapted from Niebyl JR. Treating breast infections. *Cont Ob/Gyn* 1996; 41(2):11-12.

NEONATAL RESUSCITATION

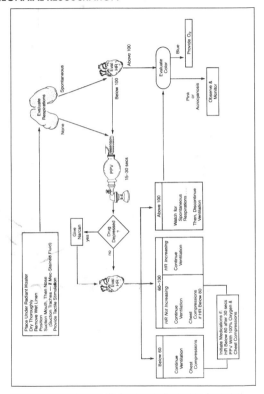

OBSTETRICS

INFANT CPR

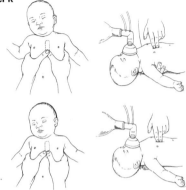

Source: Schuman AJ. Neonatal resuscitation: what you need to know. *Cont Ob/Gyn* 1992;37(12):96. Reproduced with the permission of the publisher, Medical Economics Publishing: Montvale, N.J.

Apgar scores

Feature	0	1	2
Appearance	blue, pale	body pink, extremities blue	pink
Pulse	absent	< 100 beats/min	> 100 beats/min
Grimace (tone)	none	grimace	cough, sneeze
Activity	limp	some tone	active
Respirations	absent	crying	good cry

Neonatal Drug Doses

Drug	Dose
Epinephrine	(1:10,000) 0.2 ml/kg IV or ET. Give rapidly. Dilute 1:1 with saline for ET use.
Volume Expansion	(whole blood, saline, 5% albumin, LR) 10 ml/kg, give over 5-10 minutes.
NaHCO₃	(0.5 mEq/ml) 1-2 mEq/kg IV. Give slowly, only if ventilation adequate.
Naloxone	(0.4 mg/ml) 0.1 mg/kg = 0.25 ml/kg IV, ET, IM, SQ. Give rapidly
Glucose	D10W 2 ml/kg IV. Give over 1-2 minutes.

Source: Baker ER, Shephrd B. Neonatal resuscitation & care of the newborn at risk. In: DeCherney AH, Pernoll ML, ed. *Current Obstetric & Gynecologic Diagnosis & Treatment.* 8th ed. Norwalk, Conn.: Appleton & Lange, 1994. Reproduced with the permission of the publisher.

ANTEPARTUM TESTING
The Biophysical Profile (BPP)

Feature	Definition
Reactive FHR:	At least two episodes of acceleration > 15 bpm lasting at least 15 seconds in a 20 minute period of monitoring.
Fetal Breathing Movement:	At least one episode of FBM of 30 sec duration in 30 minutes.
Gross Body Movements:	At least 3 discrete body/limb movements in 30 minutes (episodes of continuous active movement considered single movement).
Fetal Tone:	At least one episode of active extension with return to flexion of limbs or trunk. Opening and closing of hand considered normal tone.
Qualitative AFV:	At least one pocket of AF that measures 2 cm in 2 perpendicular planes. Normal AFI > 8 cm, oligo < 5, equivocal 5-8, polyhydramnios > 20.
Bradycardia:	A decrease from the baseline of at least 40 beats per minute, or an absolute heart rate of 90 bpm or less, lasting ≥ 60 seconds.

Source: Adapted from Manning FA et al. Antepartum fetal evaluation: development of a fetal biophysical profile score. *Am J Obstet Gynecol.* 1980; 136:787. Reproduced wth permission.

BPP Management

BPP Score	Interpretation	Risk of Asphyxia* (%)	Risk of Fetal Death (per 1,000/week)	Recommended Management
10/10 8/10 (normal AFI) 8/8 (NST not done)	Nonasphyxiated	0	0.565	No Indication for intervention for fetal indications
8/10 (oligo)	Chronic compensated asphyxia	5-10 (estimate)	20-30	If mature (≥ 37 weeks) deliver. Serial testing (twice weekly) in the immature fetus.
6/10 (normal AFI)	Acute asphyxia possible	10	50	If mature (≥ 37 weeks) deliver. Repeat testing in 24 hours in the immature fetus. If repeat testing 6/10 then deliver.
6/10 (oligo)	Chronic asphyxia with possible acute asphyxia	>10	>50	Factor in gestational age. If 32 weeks then deliver. If ≤ 32 weeks, test daily.
4/10 (normal AFI)	Acute asphyxia likely	36	115	Factor in gestational age. If 32 weeks then deliver. If ≤ 32 weeks, test daily.
4/10 (oligo)	Chronic asphyxia, acute asphyxia likely	>36	>115	If ≥ 26 weeks deliver.
2/10 (normal AFV)	Acute asphyxia nearly certain	73	220	If ≥ 26 weeks deliver.
2/10 (oligo)	Chronic asphyxia with superimposed acute asphyxia	>73	>220	If ≥ 26 weeks deliver.
0/10	Gross severe asphyxia	100	550	If ≥ 26 weeks deliver.

*umbilical venous metabolic acidosis < 7.25

Source: Adapted from Manning FA. Fetal Biophysical Profile. *Obstet Gynecol Clinics NA* 1999,26:557-577. Reproduced wth permission.

OBSTETRICS

ANTENATAL TESTING GUIDELINES

Condition	Timing of Testing	Test and Frequency
Diabetes Mellitus		
diet-controlled with no complications	34 wk - delivery	NST q week
insulin-dependent in good control	34 wk - delivery	NST q week
diet-controlled with previous IUFD and/or other medical problem	26 wk - 32 wk	NST q week
insulin-dependent with poor control	32 wk - delivery	NST 2x week
previous IUFD	at ≥ 40 weeks	NST 2x week and BPP

Good control = pregestational diabetic in good control prior to 12 weeks, or GDM in good control before 32 weeks.

Post dates / poor dates using earliest EDC		
	40 - 40.6 weeks	NST q week
	41 - 41.6 weeks	NST 2x week and AFI
	≥ 42 weeks	NST 3x week, BPP at 42 wk

Delivery is often advocated at ≥ 42 weeks, but if the delivery option is not chosen, observe the above protocol.
Normal NST, CST, BPP with low or very low AFI -> consider delivery

Multiple mild variables (>3 in 5 min) or any lasting > 30 sec		
		perform AFI -> frequency of subsequent testing on case by case basis

Assorted Clinical Problems		
abnormal FHT's by auscultation	26 weeks or at onset of problem	NST q week
asthma (with hypoxia)		
cardiac disease		
cholestasis of pregnancy		
collagen vascular disease - in remission		
congenital anomalies		
decreased fetal movement		
late prenatal care (3rd trimester) 1 test only if normal		
multiple gestation		
oligohydramnios		
placenta previa - no bleeding		
polyhydramnios		
thyroid disease		
poor OB history		
preterm labor		
PUBS or IUT		
renal disease		
Rh disease		
sickle cell disease (daily in crisis)		
previous IUFD		
third trimester bleeding		
chronic HTN		NST 2x week
preeclampsia		
IUGR		
PROM		

ANTENATAL TESTING GUIDELINES (CONT)

The Premature Fetus
• baseline heart rate never < 100 or > 160
• reactivity occurs after 20 weeks
• decels may be predictive of fetal compromise in some clinical situations

Gestational Age	% Reactive
20 - 24 weeks	30%
24 - 28 weeks	50%
28 - 30 weeks	75%
30 - 32 weeks	85%
32 - 36 weeks	98%

Source: Druzin ML, Fox A, Kogut E, Carlson C. The relationship of the nonstress test to gestational age. *Am J Obstet Gynecol* 1985; 153:386.

Decision Tree

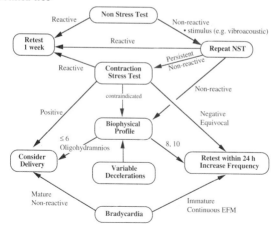

OBSTETRICS

ASTHMA IN PREGNANCY

Fast Facts
- no predictable effect on asthma
- 1/3 improved, 1/3 worsened, 1/3 unchanged
- mild asthmatics at low risk
- severe asthmatics should have high-risk follow-up
- mortality of asthma is that of mechanical ventilatory fatigue

Evaluation
- oxygen consumption increases 25% in pregnancy
- pCO_2 normally falls in pregnancy
- non-pregnant normal $PaCO_2$ levels may signal severe CO_2 retention in pregnancy

Therapy-Chronic Outpatient

Drug Class	Specific Drug	Dosage
Anti-inflammatory	Cromolyn sodium	2 puffs qid (inhalation) 2 sprays in each nostril bid (for nasal symptoms)
	Beclomethasone	2-5 puffs bid-qid (inhalation) 2 sprays in each nostril bid (intranasal for allergic rhinitis)
	Prednisone	Burst for active symptoms: 40 mg/day for 1 week then taper for 1 week; if prolonged course required single AM dose on alternative days may minimize adverse effects
Bronchodilator	Inhaled beta$_2$-agonist	2 puffs every 4 hours as needed
	Theophylline	Oral: dose to reach serum concentration level of 8-12 mcg/mL
Antihistamine	Chlorpheniramine	4 mg orally up to qid 8-12 mg sustained release bid
	Tripelennamine	25-50 mg orally up to qid 100 mg sustained release bid
Decongestant	Pseudoephedrine	60 mg orally up to qid 120 mg sustained release bid
	Oxymetazoline	Intranasal spray or drops up to 5 days for rhinosinusitis
Cough	Guaifenesin Dextromethorphan	2 tsp orally qid
Antibiotics	Amoxicillin	3 weeks therapy for sinusitis

ASTHMA IN PREGNANCY (CONT.)
Asthma in Pregnancy-Acute Management (Emergency Room)

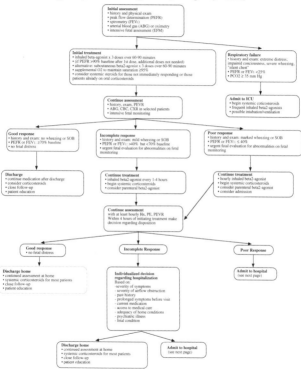

Initial assessment
• history and physical exam
• peak flow determination (PEFR)
• spirometry (FEV1)
• arterial blood gas (ABG) or oximetry
• intensive fetal assessment (EFM)

Initial treatment
• inhaled beta-agonist x 3 doses over 60-90 minutes
• (if PEFR >90% baseline after 1st dose, additional doses not needed)
• alternative: subcutaneous beta2-agonist x 3 doses over 60-90 minutes
• supplemental O2 to maintain saturation ≥95%
• consider systemic steroids for those not immediately responding or those patients already on oral corticosteroids

Respiratory failure
• hoiory and exam: extreme distress; impaired conciousness, severe wheezing, "silent chest"
• PEFR or FEV1 <25%
• PCO2 ≥ 35 mm Hg

Admit to ICU
• begin systemic corticosteroids
• frequent inhaled beta2-agonists
• possible intubation/ventilation

Continue assessment
• history, exam, PEVR
• ABG, CBC, CXR in selected patients
• intensive fetal monitoring

Good response
• history and exam: no wheezing or SOB
• PEFR or FEV1: ≥70% baseline
• no fetal distress

Incomplete response
• history and exam: mild wheezing or SOB
• PEFR or FEV1: ≥40% but <70% baseline
• urgent fetal evaluation for abnormalities on fetal monitoring

Poor response
• history and exam: marked wheezing or SOB
• PEFR or FEV1: ≤ 40%
• urgent fetal evaluation for abnormalities on fetal monitoring

Discharge
• continue medication after discharge
• consider corticosteroids
• close follow-up
• patient education

Continue treatment
• inhaled beta2-agonist every 1-4 hours
• begin systemic corticosteroids
• consider parenteral beta2-agonist

Continue treatment
• hourly inhaled beta2-agonist
• begin systemic corticosteroids
• consider parenteral beta2-agonist
• consider admission

Continue assessment
with at least hourly Ha, PE, PEVR
Within 4 hours of initiating treatment make decision regarding disposition

Good response
• no fetal distress

Incomplete Response

Poor Response

Discharge home
• continued assessment at home
• systemic corticosteroids for most patients
• close follow-up
• patient education

Individualized decision regarding hospitalization
Based on:
- severity of symptoms
- severity of airflow obstruction
- past history
- prolonged symptoms before visit
- current medication
- access to medical care
- adequacy of home conditions
- psychiatric illness
- fetal condition

Admit to hospital
(see next page)

Discharge home
• continued assessment at home
• systemic corticosteroids for most patients
• close follow-up
• patient education

Admit to hospital
(see next page)

Source: *Report of the Working Group on Asthma and Pregnancy.* Management of Asthma During Pregnancy. NIH Publication No. 93-3279, September 1993.

OBSTETRICS

ASTHMA IN PREGNANCY (CONT.)

Asthma in Pregnancy-Acute Management (Hospital)

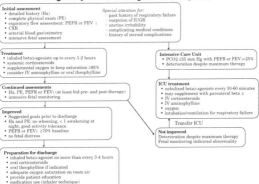

Initial assessment
- detailed history (Hx)
- complete physical exam (PE)
- expiratory flow assessment: PEFR or FEV₁
- CXR
- arterial blood gas/oximetry
- intensive fetal assessment

Special attention for:
- past history of respiratory failure
- suspicion of IUGR
- uterine irritability
- complicating medical conditions
- history of steroid complications

Treatment
- inhaled beta2-agonists up to every 1-2 hours
- systemic corticosteroids
- supplemental oxygen to keep saturation ≥95%
- consider IV aminophylline or oral theophylline

Continued assessments
- Hx, PE, PEFR or FEV₁ (at least bid pre- and post-therapy)
- intensive fetal monitoring

Improved
- Suggested goals prior to discharge
- Hx and PE: no wheezing, < 1 awakening at night, good activity tolerance
- PEFR or FEV₁ ≥70% baseline
- no fetal distress

Preparation for discharge
- inhaled beta2-agonist no more than every 3-4 hours
- oral corticosteroids
- oral theophylline if indicated
- adequate oxygen saturation on room air
- provide patient education
- medication use (inhaler technique)
- PEFR measurements at home
- need for follow-up within 7-10 days

Intensive Care Unit
- PCO₂ ≥35 mm Hg with PEFR or FEV₁ <25%
- deterioration despite maximum therapy

ICU treatment
- nebulized beta2-agonists every 30-60 minutes
- may supplement with parenteral beta 2
- IV corticosteroids
- IV aminophylline
- oxygen
- intubation/ventilation for respiratory failure

Transfer ICU

Not improved
Deterioration despite maximum therapy
Fetal monitoring indicated abnormality

Source: *Report of the Working Group on Asthma and Pregnancy.* Management of Asthma During Pregnancy. NIH Publication No. 93-3279, September 1993.

Drug Class	Specific Drug	Dosage
Beta-Agonists		
Inhaled	Albuterol	albuterol 2.5 mg (0.5 cc of a 0.5% solution, diluted with 2-3 cc of normal saline)
	Metaproterenol	metaproterenol 15 mg (0.3 cc of a 5% solution, diluted with 2-3 cc of normal saline)
Subcutaneous	Terbutaline	0.25 mg
Methylxanthines		
Intravenous	Theophylline	intravenous loading dose: theophylline 5 mg/kg intravenous maintenance dose: theophylline 0.4 mg/kg/hr
	Aminophylline	intravenous loading dose: aminophylline 6 mg/kg intravenous maintenance dose: aminophylline 0.5 mg/kg/hr,
Corticosteroids		
Intravenous	Methylprednisolone	1 mg/kg IV bolus every 6-8 hours
	Hydrocortisone	2.0 mg/kg IV bolus every 4 hours or 2.0 mg/kg IV bolus then 0.5 mg/kg/hr continuous infusion
Oral	Prednisone or methylprednisolone	prednisone or methylprednisolone 60 mg then 60-120 mg/day in divided doses, tapered over several days*

* With improvements in the patient's condition corticosteroids are usually tapered to a single daily dose or divided doses and gradually reduced over 7-14 days. Side effects may be minimized in those patients on prolonged courses of oral corticosteroids by using single AM doses on alternating days.

GESTATIONAL DIABETES

Screening for Gestational Diabetes

• use either a two-step screening with initial 50 g GCT followed by a diagnostic OGTT or eliminate the GCT and screen all appropriate patients with OGTT
• GCT = non-fasting 50 g oral glucose challenge test
    • venous plasma glucose measured one hour later
    • value of ≥140 mg/dL indicates need for 3 hour OGTT (~80% sensitivity)
    • value of ≥130 mg/dL will improve sensitivity to 90% but will necessitate OGTT on 25% of women

Risk Category	Recommendations for Screening
High risk (one or more of the following)	
Marked obesity Diabetes in first degree relative History of glucose intolerance Previous infant with macrosomia Current glycosuria	Screen at initial antepartum visit or as soon as possible; repeat at 24-28 weeks gestation if initial screening negative for gestational diabetes
Average risk	
Patient fits neither the high-risk nor low-risk profile.	Screen between 24 and 28 weeks gestation
Low risk (all of the following)	
Age < 25 years Belongs to a low-risk race or ethnic group‡ No diabetes in first degree relative Normal prepregnancy weight and weight gain during pregnancy No history of abnormal blood glucose levels No prior poor obstetrical outcomes	Not required

‡ Low-risk races and ethnic groups are those other than Hispanic, black, Native American, South or East Asian, Pacific Islander or Indigenous Australian

Source: Kjos SL and Buchanan TA. Gestational Diabetes Mellitus. *N Engl J Med* 1999;341(23):1749-1756. Reproduced with permission of the Massachusetts Medical Society.

Diagnosis of Gestational Diabetes

• 100 g oral glucose load administered after overnight fast
• test should be given after 3 days of unrestricted diet (>150 g of carbohydrates/day) and activity
• venous plasma glucose is measured at fasting, 1 hr, 2 hr and 3 hr
• two or more abnormal values = gestational diabetes

Fasting	95 mg/dL
1 hour	180 mg/dL
2 hour	155 mg/dL
3 hour	140 mg/dL

OBSTETRICS

GESTATIONAL DIABETES (CONT.)

Management
• for an excellent review see Metzger BE, Coustan DR et al. Summary and Recommendations of the Fourth International Workshop-Conference on Gestational Diabetes Mellitus. *Diabetes Care* 1998;21 Supp 2, B161-B168.

Diet (Body Mass Index more exact)
• Ideal Body Weight (IBW) = 100 lb @ 5 feet, plus 5 lb/inch > 5 ft
• Daily kcal: 36 kcal/kg or 15 kcal/lb of IBW + 100 kcal/trimester
• Nutrients
    • 40-50% carbohydrate
    • 12-20% protein
    • 30-35% fat

Glucose Monitoring
• Desired ranges

California Diabetes in Pregnancy Program
    "Sweet Success"
    Fasting 70-105 mg/dL
    2 hr post-prandial 100-140 mg/dL

Others
    Fasting 60-90 mg/dL
    Premeal 60-105 mg/dL
    After Meal ≤ 120 mg/dL
    2AM - 4AM 60 mg/dL

Insulin
• usually begun for fastings > 105 mg/dL consistently
• anticipated eventual insulin requirements for gestational diabetic listed below
• distribution
    A.M. 2/3 → 2/3 NPH, 1/3 Reg
    P.M. 1/3 → 1/2 NPH, 1/2 Reg
• IDDM require individualization (see following page)

Gestational Age (weeks)	Anticipated Insulin Dose
6-18	0.7 Units/kg
18-26	0.8 Units/kg
26-36	0.9 Units/kg
36-40	1.0 Units/kg

Type of Insulin	Onset of Action	Maximum Effect	Duration
Regular	1 hour	2-3 hours	4-5 hours
NPH	2 hours	8 hours	24 hours
PZI	4 hours		36 hours

INSULIN DEPENDENT DIABETES AND PREGNANCY

Management of Insulin Dependent Diabetics in Pregnancy

- √ HgB $_{A1C}$ preconception and during 1st trimester
  - rate of malformations 22% for HgB $_{A1C}$ > 8.5
- fetal cardiac echocardiogram at 22 weeks
- ophthalmology evaluation during 1st and 3rd trimesters
- 24 hour urine for creatinine clearance, total protein
- ultrasound at 18, 22, 26, 38 weeks; consider amnio for maturity at 38 weeks
- consider primary cesarean if EFW > 4000 g (see section on shoulder dystocia, page 31)
- √ blood sugar q 2 hr in labor and if > 120 start insulin drip (10 U in 1000 cc) to keep BS 85-100 mg/dL
- if elective cesarean, then give AM insulin, perform AM Cesarean

DKA During Pregnancy

Evaluation	Therapy
Laboratory assessment	Arterial blood gas, then glucose, ketones, electrolytes q 2 hr
Insulin	Low dose, intravenous Regular insulin Loading dose: 0.2 - 0.4 Units/kg Maintenance 2.0 - 10 Units/hr
Fluids	Isotonic NaCl Total replacement in first 12 hr = 4-6 liters 500-1000 mL/hr for 2-4 hours 250 mL/hr until 80% replaced
Glucose	Begin D5-NS when plasma glucose reaches 250 mg/dL
Potassium	If initially normal or reduced then add 40-60 mEq/L If initially elevated then give 20-30 mEq/L once levels begin to decline
Bicarbonate	Add one amp (44 mEq) to 1 L of 0.45 NS if pH is < 7.10

Source: Landon MB. Diabetes mellitus and other endocrine diseases. In: Gabbe SG, Niebyl JR, Simpson JL, ed. *Obstetrics: Normal and Problem Pregnancies.* 2nd ed. New York: Churchill Livingstone, 1991. Reproduced with the permission of the publisher.

White Classification

Class	Onset	Duration	Vascular Disease
A	any	any	None
B	> 20 years old	< 10 years	None
C	10-19 years old	10-19 years	None
D	≤ 10 years old	≥ 20 years	Benign retinopathy
EF	Any	Any	Nephropathy
R	Any	Any	Proliferative retinopathy
H	Any	Any	Heart disease
RT	Any	Any	Renal transplant

GDM		
A-1	Fasting < 105 mg/dL; Postprandial < 120 mg/dL Diet controlled	
A-2	Fasting ≤ 105 mg/dL; Postprandial > 120 mg/dL Insulin requiring	

OBSTETRICS

CLASSIFICATION OF HYPERTENSIVE DISORDERS OF PREGNANCY
Chronic Hypertension
• hypertension present and observable before pregnancy or prior to 20th week of gestaton
• hypertension defined as blood pressure > 140 mm Hg systolic or 90 mm Hg diastolic

Preeclampsia-Eclampsia
• hypertension defined as blood pressure > 140 mm Hg systolic or 90 mm Hg diastolic in a previously
    normotensive patient
• previous incremental rise in blood pressure has not been included but rise in blood pressure of 30 mm
    Hg systolic or 15 mm Hg diastolic warrants close observation
• proteinuria of 300 mg in 24 hours
• findings that increase the certainty of the diagnosis include:
    • blood pressure of >160 mm Hg systolic or >110 mm Hg diastolic
    • proteinuria of > 2 g in 24 hr (should occur for the first time in pregnancy)
    • increased serum creatinine (>1.2 mg/dL unless previously known to be elevated)
    • platelet count < 100,000 cells/mm^3 and/or evidence of microangiopathic hemolytic anemia
    • elevated hepatic enzymes (AST and ALT)
    • persistent headache or other cerebral or visual disturbances
    • persistent epigastric pain
• eclampsia is the occurence of seizures in a woman with preeclampsia (unattributed to other causes)
• edema has been abandoned as a marker

Preeclampsia Superimposed upon Chronic Hypertension
• prognosis worse than in either condition alone
• overdiagnosis is appropriate and unavoidable
• consider this diagnosis in following findings:
    • new onset proteinuria (300 mg/24 hr) in a hypertensive woman without previous proteinuria
    • hypertension and proteinuria prior to 20 weeks gestation
    • sudden increase in proteinuria
    • sudden increase in blood pressure in a previously well-controlled patient
    • platelet count < 100,000 cells/mm^3
    • elevated hepatic enzymes (AST and ALT)

Gestational Hypertension
• used until a more specific diagnosis can be assigned
• may represent preeclampsia prior to proteinuria or chronic hypertension previously unrecognized

Source: *National High Blood Pressure Education Program Working Group Report on High Blood Pressure in Pregnancy,*
NIH Publication No. 00-3029, July 2000.

MANAGEMENT OF PIH

Source: National High Blood Pressure Education Program Working Group Report on High Blood Pressure in Pregnancy, NIH Publication No. 00-3029, July 2000.

Laboratory Evaluation

Test	Rationale
Hemoglobin and hematocrit	Hemoconcentration supports the diagnosis of preeclampsia and is an indicator of severity. Values may be decreased, however, if hemolysis accompanies the disease.
Platelet count	Thrombocytopenia suggests preeclampsia.
Quantification of protein excretion	Pregnancy hypertension with proteinuria should be considered preeclampsia (pure or superimposed) until it is proven otherwise.
Serum creatinine level	Abnormal or rising creatinine levels, especially in association with oliguria, suggest severe preeclampsia.
Serum uric acid level	Increased uric acid levels suggest the diagnosis of preeclampsia.
Serum transaminase levels	Rising serum transaminase levels suggest severe preeclampsia with hepatic involvement.
Serum albumin, lactic acid dehydrogenase, blood smear and coagulation profile	For women with severe disease, these values indicate the extent of endothelial leak (hypoalbuminemia), presence of hemolysis (LDH level, peripheral smear) and possible coagulopathy including thrombocytopenia.

Hypertensive Emergency
(BP > 160 mm HG systolic or > 105 mm Hg diastolic)

Drug	Administration
Hydralazine	Start with 5 mg IV or 10 mg IM. If blood pressure is not controlled, repeat at 20-minute intervals (5 to 10 mg depending on response). Once blood pressure is controlled repeat as needed (usually about 3 hours). If no success by 20 mg IV or 30 mg IM total, consider another drug.
Labetalol	Start with 20 mg IV as a bolus; if effect is suboptimal, then give 40 mg 10 minutes later and 80 mg every 10 minutes for two additional doses. Use a maximum of 220 mg. If desired blood pressure levels are not achieved, switch to another drug. Do not give labetalol to women with asthma or congestive heart failure.
Nifedipine	Start with 10 mg orally and repeat in 30 minutes if necessary. Short acting nifedipine is NOT approved by the FDA for managing hypertension. Refer to the Working Group Report for details.
Sodium nitroprusside	Rarely needed for hypertension not responding to the drugs listed above and/or if there are clinical findings of hypertensive encephalopathy. Start at a rate of 0.25 mcg/kg/min to a maximum of 5 mcg/kg/min. Fetal cyanide poisoning may occur if used for more than 4 hours.

Caution: Sudden and severe hypotension can result from the administration of any of these agents, especially short-acting oral nifedipine. The goal of blood pressure reduction in emergency situations should be a gradual reduction of blood pressure to the normal range.

Indications for Delivery

Maternal	Fetal
Gestational age 38 weeks	Severe fetal growth restriction
Platelet count < 100,000 cells/mm3	Nonreassuring fetal testing results
Progressive deterioration in hepatic function	Oligohydramnios
Progressive deterioration in renal function	
Suspected abruptio placentae	
Persistent severe headaches or visual changes	
Persistent severe epigastric pain, nausea or vomiting	

Delivery should be based on maternal and fetal conditions as well as gestational age

OBSTETRICS

MANAGEMENT OF PIH (CONT.)
Mild Preeclampsia
• deliver if at term
• if premature then hospitalize
  • √ NST's, PIH symptoms, weight gain, urine output, urine dipsticks
  • initial labs (hematocrit uric acid, platelets, SGOT, fibrinogen, creatinine)
  • begin 24 hr urine collection
  • deliver if meet criteria for severe
• begin MgSO₄ seizure prophylaxis when in labor or at time of induction
  • 4 g IV load then 2 g IV per hour, watch level if decreased renal function

Severe Preeclampsia
• delivery indicated for maternal health
• occasionally will not declare as severe for 1-2 days
  • consider β-methasone for fetal lung maturity
• consider primary cesarean if primigravida, unfavorable cervix and < 32 wks EGA
• fluid restrict 2400 cc/24 hr
• watch urine output (oliguria < 30 cc/hr), Swan-Ganz may be helpful
• monitor pulmonary status closely
• monitor for fetal distress (often subtle late decels)
• begin MgSO₄ for seizure prophylaxis
• monitor lab closely (platelets, Mg⁺² level, LFT's)
• keep diastolic blood pressure 90-105 mm Hg with hydralazine or labetolol
• if pulmonary edema → treat aggressively with furosemide
  • some maternal deaths are secondary to pulmonary edema

HELLP Syndrome
• delivery indicated
• treat as severe preeclampsia

MgSO₄ Overdose	
Toxicity - 1 gram Ca⁺² gluconate IV push	
EKG changes	5-10 mEq/liter
Loss of deep tendon reflexes	10 mEq/liter
Respiratory suppression	15 mEq/liter
Cardiovascular collapse	>25 mEq/liter

Eclampsia
• ABC
  • administer O₂
  • oral airway if decreased consciousness
  • place lines
  • place Foley
  • consider Swan-Ganz (CVP alone often inadequate)
• fetal monitoring after the seizure
• MgSO₄ 4-6 g IV loading dose then 2 g/hr
  • reload for recurrent seizure
• consider Valium 10 mg IV push if seizes again

Postpartum
• continue MgSO₄ for 24 hr or until diuresis begins
• watch BP, pulmonary status closely, continue fluid restriction
• follow labs as indicated
• treat BP as needed, limit crystalloid fluid challenges with low urine output
• early return to clinic if BP still elevated

INTRAUTERINE FETAL DEMISE (IUFD) EVALUATION

1. Confirm by ultrasound (2 examiners)
2. Maternal blood work
   - Hgb $_{A1C}$
   - Kleihauer-Betke
   - RPR (VDRL)
   - FANA, PTT, anti-cardiolipin antibodies
   - serum/urine toxicology screen
3. Fetal evaluations
   - chromosomes
   - cord blood/cardiac puncture (in green-top tube-heparinized)
   - skin biopsy (in normal saline)
   - genetics evaluation (dysmorphology)
   - autopsy
4. Placental pathology evaluation
5. Grief and loss follow-up

NON-IMMUNE HYDROPS EVALUATION

Ultrasound	Maternal Blood
Placenta	3 hour OGTT
hemangioma	Type and screen
thickened	Kleihauer-Betke
triploidy syndromes	AFP
maternal diabetes	G-6-PD
fetal anemia	CMV, toxo, parvovirus B19 titers
thin (dysmaturity)	VDRL
Umbilical cord	Rheumatoid factor, anti-nuclear antibody (ANA)
thrombus	BUN, creatinine, uric acid
Amniotic fluid	mirror syndrome
polyhydramnios (usual)	• preeclampsia type maternal illness associated with fetal hydrops
oligohydramnios (with triploidy)	
Fetus	
ascites, pleural effusion, pericardial effusion	
edema	
twin-twin transfusion	
fetal sex (G-6-PD deficiency)	
enlarged heart, cardiac tumor	
fetal bradycardia (heart block)	
pulmonary hypoplasia	
cystic adenomatoid malformation of lung	
diaphragmatic hernia	
sacrococcygeal teratoma	
short-limbed dwarfism	
cystic hygroma	
alpha thalassemia	

OBSTETRICS

ISOIMMUNIZATION

Maternal Type and Screen
- Antibody screen negative
  - Determine Rh status
    - If D neg and father D positive or unknown
      - Repeat screen at 28 wks offer RhoGam if negative
    - If D positive no further eval
- Antibody screen positive
  - Screen father for antigen status
    - Negative for antigen
      - No further evaluation
    - Positive for antigen or unknown
      - Maternal titer and detailed history

Titers apply only to anti-D

Titer ≤ 1:32
- Follow Maternal titers starting at 16-18 wks, q 2-4 wks
  - Liley zone I, lower zone II, USG normal
    - Deliver at or near term
  - Upper zone II
    - PUBS or repeat amnio in 1 wk
  - Liley zone III, hydramnios, hydrops
    - <32-34 wks
      - IUT
    - >32-34 wks
      - Delivery

Titer > 1:32
- After 27 wks, monitor with serial amnio, USG
  - Before 27 wks, timing of initial dx procedure secondary to OB hx, USG and titer elevation
    - Good OB hx, titer < 1:64, USG normal
      - Serial amnios and USG q 2 wks
    - Poor OB hx, titer > 1:64 or hydramnios
      - PUBS for Hct type
        - Antigen positive, fetus anemic
        - Antigen positive, fetus not anemic
          - Monitor with PUBS, interval secondary to OB hx, USG, last Hct
            - Fetus anemic
              - IUT
            - Fetus not anemic
        - Antigen negative
          - No further evaluation

From American College of Obstetricians and Gynecologists: *Management of Isoimmunization in Pregnancy.* Technical Bulletin 148. ACOG, Washington, DC © 1990. Reproduced with the permission of the publisher.

LILEY CURVE

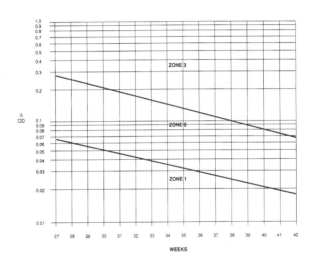

From Liley AW. Liquor amnii analysis in management of pregnancy complicated by Rhesus sensitization. *Am J Obstet Gynecol* 1961;82(6):1359. Reproduced with the permission of the publisher, Mosby-Year Book: St. Louis.

OBSTETRICS

MULTIPLE GESTATION

Fast Facts
- Dizygotic: fertilization of 2 separate ova by 2 sperm
- Monozygotic: division of single ovum fertilized by single sperm
- incidence: MZ 4/1000 worldwide, DZ 8/1000 in U.S., 41/1000 in Nigeria
- twins account for < 1% deliveries but 10% of perinatal mortality
- 75% of twins show some evidence of growth abnormalities
  - 25-30% meet criteria for IUGR
- average length of gestation
  - twins   35 weeks (36% deliver < 34 wks, 50% deliver < 37 wks)
  - triplets   33 weeks
  - quads   29 weeks

Placentation
- Dizygotic twins have separate chorion/amnion (2/3 of U.S. twins)
- Monozygotic twins dependent on division (1/3 of U.S. twins)

0-72 hr	diamniotic, dichorionic (30%)
4-8 d	monochorionic, diamniotic (68%)
8-13 d	monochorionic, monoamniotic (2%)
> 13 d	conjoined twins

Maternal Complications
- hyperemesis
- PIH
- pyelonephritis
- post-partum hemorrhage
- preterm labor

Antepartum Management
- high risk for preterm labor
- serial USG for growth
- NST as indicated
  - may be useful in multiple gestations to assess fetal well-being and predict cord compression

Presentation

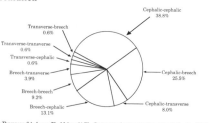

Source: Thompson SA, Lyons TL, Makowski EL. Outcomes of twin gestations at the University of Colorado Health Sciences Center, 1973-1983. *J Reprod Med* 1987;32(5):328-39. Reproduced with the permission of the publisher, the Journal of Reproductive Medicine.

MULTIPLE GESTATION DELIVERY
Presentation
- vertex/vertex 40%
- vertex/non-vertex 40%
- non-vertex/other 20%

Management

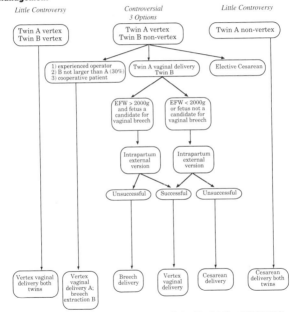

Source: Chervenak FA, Johnson RE, Youcha S, et al. Intrapartum management of twin gestation. *Obstet Gynecol* 1985;65(1):119-24.
Reproduced with the permission of the publisher, the American College of Obstetricians and Gynecologists.

OBSTETRICS

PRETERM LABOR

Fast Facts

- Preterm birth represents greatest source of perinatal morbidity and mortality
- Spontaneous preterm labor (50%)
- Indicated preterm delivery (20%)
- Preterm premature rupture of membranes (PPROM) (30%)

Diagnosis:

1. Estimated gestational age < 36 completed weeks
2. Uterine activity
3. Cervical dilation > 2 cm or 80% effaced
4. Documented cervical change from single examiner

Principles of Management (outpatient)

- Weekly cervical exams (20-37 weeks)
- Home self-monitoring
- Pelvic rest
- Bedrest
- Early intervention for cervical change
- Education
- Identification of high risk patients

Prevention

- Home uterine activity monitoring of unproven benefit
- Fetal fibronectin screening may be predictive of preterm delivery
  - negative predictive value between 24-34 weeks
- Cervical length on sonogram may be predictive of preterm delivery
- Antibiotic therapy for bacterial vaginosis may be helpful in "at-risk" patients
- Prophylactic treatment of mother for Group B streptococcus is appropriatepending culture results
- Tocolytic therapy may at least provide for administration of corticosteroids or transport to tertiary center for delivery

First Birth	Second Birth	Number	Subsequent Preterm Birth	
			Percent	Relative Risk
Term	-------	25,814	4.4	1.0
Preterm	-------	1,860	17.2	3.9
Term	Term	1,540	5.7	1.3
Preterm	Term	1,128	11.1	2.5
Preterm	Preterm	320	28.4	6.5

Source: Bakketeig LS, Hoffman HJ. Epidemiology of preterm birth: results from a longitudinal study of births in Norway. In: Elder LS, Hendricks CH, eds. *Preterm Labor.* London/Boston: Butterworths; 1981:17-46.

PRETERM LABOR (CONT)

Maternal Characteristics Associated with Increased Risk

- History of previous preterm birth
- Maternal race (more black than nonblack)
- Poor nutrition/low body mass index
- Low socioeconomic status
- Absent or inadequate prenatal care
- Age < 18 or > 40 years
- Strenuous work
- High personal stress
- Cigarette smoking
- Anemia (hemoglobin < 10 g/dL)
- Bacteriuria
- Genital colonization or infection (eg, bacterial vaginosis, *Neisseria gonorrhea, Chlamydia trachomatis,* Mycoplasma and Ureaplasma)
- Cervical injury or abnormalitiy (eg, in utero exposure to diethylstilbesterol, history of cervical conization, second trimester induced abortion)
- Uterine anomaly or fibroids
- Excessive uterine contractility
- Premature cervical dilation (>1 cm) or effacement (~80%)

Source: APGO Educational Series on Women's Health Issues: *Prevention and Management of Preterm Birth.* © 1998 Association of Professors of Gynecology and Obstetrics. Washington, DC.

Risk Factors for Preterm Delivery and PPROM

Risk Factor	Preterm PROM	Preterm Delivery Without PROM
Prior preterm delivery	6.3 (1.9-21)	21.3 (4-105)
Smoking	4.9 (1.5-6.8)	2.9 (0.6-12)
Bleeding		
First trimester	0.8 (0.2-2.4)	1.8 (0.2-13)
Second trimester	15.1 (2.8-81)	19.7 (2.1-186)
Third trimester	4.6 (0.9-23)	1.5 (0.4-5.4)

Source: Ekwo EE, Gosselink CA, Moawad A. Unfavorable outcome in penultimate pregnancy and premature rupture of the membranes in successive pregnancy. *Obstet Gynecol.* 1992;80:166-172.

OBSTETRICS

ANTENATAL STEROIDS
Fast Facts
• use first described in 1972
• in spite of clear evidence supporting use only 12-18% of women delivering infants weighing 501-1500 g received steroids

Efficacy

	Quality of evidence for benefit, grade	Strength of recommendation
Interval from treatment to delivery		
< 24 hours	I	B
24 hours to 7 days	I	A
> 7 days	I	C
Gestational age		
Delivery at 24-28 weeks	I	A
Delivery at 29-34 weeks	I	A
Delivery at >34 weeks	I	C
Preterm premature rupture of membranes	I	B
Neonatal outcomes		
Mortality	I	A
Respiratory distress syndrome	I	A
Intraventricular hemorrhage	I	A

Quality of Evidence

Grade I: Evidence obtained from at least one properly designed randomized controlled trial.

Grade II-1: Evidence obtained from well designed controlled trials without randomization

Grade II-2: Evidence obtained from well designed cohort or case control analytic studies

Grade II-3: Evidence obtained from multiple time series with or without intervention.

Grade III: Opinions of respected authorities, based on clinical experience, descriptive studies, or reports of expert committees.

Strength of Recommendation

A: There is good evidence to support use.

B: There is fair evidence to support use.

C: There is inadequate evidence to argue for or against use.

D: There is fair evidence to avoid use.

E: There is good evidence to avoid use.

Dose
β-methasone
• 12 mg IM given in 2 doses 24 hours apart

Dexamethasone
• 6 mg IM given in 4 doses, one every 12 hours

Timing and Associated Therapies
• clear benefits present even if delivery occurs within 24 hours of administration
• availability of surfactant therapy should not influence decision to administer antenatal steroids
• use of thyrotropin releasing hormone (TRH) is experimental, controlled studies currently in progress

From NIH Consensus Conference. Effect of corticosteroids for fetal maturation on perinatal outcomes. *JAMA* 1995; 273(5):413. Reproduced with permission from the American Medical Association.

TOCOLYTIC AGENTS

	Contraindications	Dose	Maternal side effects	Fetal Side Effects	Monitor
Magnesium sulfate	Myasthenia gravis Impaired renal function Recent MI	Load: 4-6 g IV over 20 min Maint: 2-3 g/hr Bolus: 2-3 g over 20 min	Flushness Muscle weakness Hypotension Hyperreflexia Respiratory depression Pulmonary edema Headache	Minimal	DTR's Urine output Breath sounds Mg^{++} level (6-8 mg/dL) Fluid restrict 2400 cc/24 hr
Nifedipine	CHF Aortic stenosis Concomitant use with $MgSO_4$ • theoretical risk of elimination of treatment for Mg^{++} toxicity	Load: 10 mg SL q 20 min x 3 doses Maint: 10-20 n g PO q 4-8 hr	Hypotension Flushing Nasal congestion Tachycardia Dizziness Nausea Nervousness Bowel changes	Minimal	BP Respiratory sx's Edema
Indomethacin	Peptic ulcer disease NSAID sensitivity EGA > 30 wks Renal disease Coagulopathy	Load: 25-100 mg PR Maint: 25 mg PO q 4-6 hr Use for about 48 hours (If longer, AFI 2x/wk)	Headache GI upset Fluid retention Prolonged bleeding time Nausea and vomiting Pruritis Bowel changes	Oligohydramnios Potential ductal closure	Amniotic fluid volume
Terbutaline	Antepartum hemorrhage CV disease Hyperthyroidism Uncontrolled diabetes	SQ 0.25 mg S3 q 1-4 hr x 24 hr Total dose not >5 mg/24 hr PO: 2.5 - 7.5 mg PO q 1.5-4 hr Aim for maternal pulse: >100 Pump: 0.05-0.10 mg/hr basal rate 0.25 mg boluses	Tachycardia Tremor Palpitations Anxiety Dyspnea Pulmonary edema	Tachycardia	Baseline tests ECG, Glucose, K^+, CBC Close Monitoring 1. BP, pulse 2. Pulmonary exam 3. Fluid restrict 2400 cc/24 hr 4. Follow glucose, K^+
Ritodrine	Absolute 1. Maternal cardiac disease 2. PIH 3. Uncontrolled DM 4. Hyperthyroidism 5. Hypovolemia 6. Multiple gestation Relative 1. Diabetes 2. Chronic HTN 3. Migraine 4. Resting tachycardia	50 mcg/min, increase by 50 mcg/min q 15-20 min until ctx's cease or side effects / max dose (350 mcg/min)	Tachycardia Tremor Palpitations Anxiety Dyspnea Pulmonary edema Headache Nausea, vomiting Hypokalemia Hyperglycemia Cardiac ischemia	Tachycardia	Baseline tests ECG, Glucose, K^+, CBC Close Monitoring 1. BP, pulse 2. Pulmonary exam 3. Fluid restrict 2400 cc/24 hr 4. Follow glucose, K^+ 5. Urine output

OBSTETRICS

PRETERM PREMATURE RUPTURE OF MEMBRANES (PPROM)

Fast Facts
• PROM occurs in approximately 10% of pregnancies (8% at term)
• associated with 30% of preterm deliveries
• preterm PROM more common in lower socioeconomic classes, teenagers, smokers, single mothers, previous STD in pregnancy, prior PROM
• 90% of term and 50% of preterm patients will enter labor within 24 hours
• 85% of preterm patients will be in labor within 1 week
• clinically evident intraamniotic infection present in 13-60% of preterm PROM patients
• rate of fetal malpresentation increased
• abruptio placentae occurs in 4-12%
• risk of antenatal fetal demise 1-2%
• risk of pulmonary hypoplasia variable
     • rarely occurs if PROM after 26 weeks
• PPROM associated with amniocentesis has better outcome than spontaneous PPROM

Diagnosis
• history
• sterile speculum exam (SSE)
• pooling
• ferning
• nitrazine positive

Management
• perform SSE
• vaginal/cervical cultures
• vaginal pool for L/S, PG
• ultrasound for presentation
• evaluate for chorioamnionitis
• begin ampicillin 2 g IV q 6 hr
• NIH Consensus Conference recommends steroids if no evidence of infection and delivery not iminent with gestational age <30-32 weeks
• consider tocolysis
• antepartum testing (institution dependent)
• monitor CBC and vitals for evidence of changing status

Future pregnancies
• 21% recurrence risk
• counsel patient to avoid strenuous exercise and heavy exertional work
• counsel the patient to refrain from tobacco and other drug use
• perform a thorough nutritional evaluation including screening for anemia
• culture for *Chlamydia*, assess for bacterial vaginosis and treat positive results
• educate re:possible symptoms that may precede PPROM, including pelvic pressure/vaginal discharge
• assess cervical dilation and effacement as for preterm labor

Adapted from Regenstein AC, Main DM. Antenatal care of the patient with previous preterm premature rupture of membranes. *Obstet Gynecol Clinics NA* 1992;19(2):387.

SYSTEMIC LUPUS ERYTHEMATOSUS (SLE)

Diagnosis

(must have 4 of 11 criteria of American College of Rheumatologists)

Malar rash	Arthritis
Discoid lesions	Pleuritis or pericarditis
Photosensitivity	Oral ulcers
Proteinuria > 0.5 g/day or cellular cast	Neurologic disorder - seizure, psychosis
Hematologic	Immunologic
• anemia	• (+) LE prep
• leukopenia	• Anti double- stranded DNA
• thrombocytopenia	• Anti SM
• anemia	• False positive VDRL
	Positive FANA

Common complaints of lupus patients

• arthritis or rheumatism for > 3 months
• fingers that become cold, pale, numb, or uncomfortable in the cold
• mouth sores for ≥ 2 weeks
• prominent facial rash for > 1 month
• photosensitivity
• pleurisy
• rapid hair loss
• seizures or convulsions

Initial labs in pregnancy

• ANA screen and titer
• Anti-dsDNA
• Anti-Ro, La (SSA, SSB)
• Lupus anticoagulant
• Anticardiolipin antibodies (see below)
• C3, C4
• CH50
• chemistry panel, electrolytes
• thyroid function tests (as indicated)
• anti-platelet antibodies
• 24 hr urine for CrCl, total protein

Common lab abnormalities

• (+) ANA   > 90%
• Anti-DNA (DS)   > 80%
• Anti-DNA (SS)   50%
• Anti-SM   30%
• Anti-Ro (SSA)   25%
(associated with neonatal lupus-rash, thrombocytopenia, heart block)

Primary Antiphospholipid Syndromes (PAPS) (must have #1 and either #2, 3, or 4 below)

1. Antiphospholipid antibodies
   • anticardiolipin (ELISA)
   • lupus anticoagulant (prolonged aPTT)
   • false positive VDRL (RPR)
2. Thrombocytopenia
3. Recurrent fetal loss
   • > 2 first trimester SAB
   • 1 or more 2nd trimester losses
4. Arterial or venous thrombosis

OBSTETRICS

MANAGEMENT OF WOMEN WITH ANTIPHOSPHOLIPID ANTIBODIES

Feature	Pregnant‡	Nonpregnant
Antiphospholipid Syndrome (APS)		
APS without prior fetal death or recurrent pregnancy loss	Heparin in prophylactic doses (15,000-20,000 U of unfractionated heparin or equivalent per day) administered subcutaneously in divided doses and low-dose aspirin daily Calcium and vitamin D supplementation	Optimal management uncertain; options include no treatment or daily treatment with low-dose aspirin
APS with prior thrombosis or stroke	Heparin to achieve full anticoagulation **or** Heparin in prophylactic doses (15,000-20,000 U of unfractionated heparin or equivalent per day) administered subcutaneously in divided doses *plus* low-dose aspirin daily and calcium and vitamin D supplementation	Warfarin administered daily in doses to maintain international normalized ratio >3.0
APS without prior pregnancy loss or thrombosis	Optimal management uncertain; options include no treatment, daily treatment with low-dose aspirin, daily treatment with prophylactic doses of heparin and low-dose aspirin	Optimal management uncertain; options include no treatment or daily treatment with low-dose aspirin
Antiphospholipid Antibodies Without APS		
Lupus anticoagulant (LA) or medium-to-high positive IgG aCL	Optimal management uncertain; options include no treatment, daily treatment with low-dose aspirin, daily treatment with prophylactic doses of heparin and low-dose aspirin	Optimal management uncertain; options include no treatment or daily treatment with low-dose aspirin
Low levels of IgG aCL, only IgM aCL, only IgA aCL without LA, antiphospholipid antibodies other than LA or aCL	Optimal management uncertain; options include no treatment or daily treatment with low-dose aspirin	Optimal management uncertain; options include no treatment or daily treatment with low-dose aspirin

* The medications shown should not be used in the presence of contraindications.
‡ Close observation of mother and fetus is necessary in all cases.
The patient should be counseled in all cases regarding symptoms of thrombosis and thromboembolism.

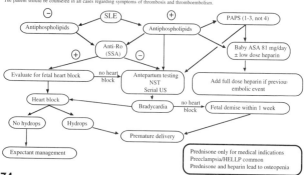

OBSTETRICS

ABRUPTIO PLACENTAE

Fast Facts
- premature separation of the normally-implanted placenta
- abruption represents 30% of third trimester bleeding
- risk factors
  - hypertension
  - cigarette smoking
  - cocaine abuse
  - trauma
  - rapid decompression of an overdistended uterus
- recurrence risk
  - 5-16%
  - increases to 25% after 2 previous abruptions
- classic signs and symptoms
  - painful vaginal bleeding
  - abdominal pain
  - uterine hypertonicity and tenderness
  - fetal distress

Management
- consider expectant management or tocolytic with mild abruption and premature fetus
- moderate to severe abruptions indicate need for delivery
- amniotomy useful in augmenting labor in anticipation of vaginal delivery
- close fetal monitoring
- perinatal mortality has been reduced by appropriate intervention with cesarean section

Grading system

Grade	Concealed hemorrhage	Uterine tenderness	Maternal shock	Coagulopathy	Fetal distress	Comments
0	No	No	Absent	No	No	Retrospective diagnosis. No symptoms.
1	No	No	Absent	No	No	Includes marginal sinus bleed, blood loss variable.
2	Yes	Yes	Absent	Rare	Yes	Usually progresses to Grade 3 unless delivered.
3	Extensive	Yes	Present	Common	Fetal death	Major maternal complications (cortical necrosis, etc.)

Source: Green JR. Placenta previa and abruptio placentae. In: Creasy RK, Resnik R, ed. *Maternal-fetal Medicine : Principles and Practice*. 3rd ed. Philadelphia: Saunders, 1994. Reproduced with the permission of the publisher.

OBSTETRICS

PLACENTA PREVIA

Fast Facts
- placenta previa represents 20% of third trimester bleeding
- incidence 1/250 live births
- bleeding is maternal
- often presents as painless, bright-red bleeding
- may be associated with contractions
- risk factors
  - previous cesarean section
  - grand multiparity

Management
- tocolytic of choice is $MgSO_4$
- no vaginal exams
- serial ultrasound for interval growth, resolution of partial previa
- delivery by cesarean
- hospitalization usually after 1st bleed, but depends on clinical situation
- consider delivery as soon as lung maturity documented
- ß-methasone (weekly injections without clinical evidence of efficacy)
- high risk for accreta, hemorrhage (especially if previous cesarean section)
  - discuss blood products, risk of hysterectomy
  - see section on uterine packing (page 41)

Evaluation

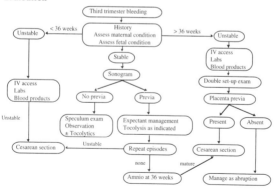

Adapted from Green JR. Placenta previa and abruptio placentae. In: Creasy RK, Resnik R, ed. *Maternal-fetal Medicine: Principles and Practice.* 3rd ed. Philadelphia: Saunders, 1994. Reproduced with the permission of the publisher.

OBSTETRICS

THROMBOEMBOLIC DISORDERS
Fast Facts
- venous thromboembolism (VTE) occurs in 0.05-0.3% of pregnancies
- monthly rates of deep vein thrombosis (DVT): 0.001% antepartum, 0.06% postpartum
  - 3-16x more common after cesarean section
- pulmonary embolism (PE) occurs in 15-24% of untreated DVT cases with mortality rate of 15%
  - PE occurs in 4.5% treated cases with mortality rate of 1%

Risk Factors for Thromboembolism

Heriditary Thrombophilia (prevalence in general population)

Factor V Leiden mutation (5-9%)*
AT-III deficiency (0.02-0.2%)
Protein C deficiency (0.2-0.5%)
Protein S deficiency (0.08%)
Hyperhomocystinemia (1-11%)
Prothrombin gene mutation G20210A (2-4%)

Prior history of deep vein thrombosis

Mechanical heart valve

Atrial fibrillation

Trauma/prolonged immobilization/major surgery

Other familial hypercoagulable states

Antiphospholipid syndrome

*For African-Americans, about 1%; for Caucasians 6-11%
Data from Lockwood CJ. Heritable coagulopathies in pregnancy. *Obstet Gynecol Surv* 1999;54:754-765.

Pregnancy Associated Changes in Coagulation
- Increases in clotting factors (I, VII, VIII, IX, X)
- Decreases in protein S
- Decreases in fibrinolytic activity
- Increased venous stasis
- Vascular injury associated with delivery
- Increased activation of platelets
- Resistance to activated protein C

Source: American College of Obstetricians and Gynecologists: *Thromboembolism in Pregnancy.* ACOG Practice Bulletin #19, August 2000. ACOG, Washington, DC © 2000. Reproduced with the permission of the publisher.

Diagnosis
- Doppler ultrasound diagnostic study of choice in proximal DVT
- ventilation-perfusion scan needed in cases of suspected pulmonary embolism
  - pulmonary angiogram may be helpful in many cases

OBSTETRICS

THROMBOEMBOLIC DISORDERS
Treatment of Pregnant Patients

Feature	Antepartum	Postpartum
Very low risk		
Varicosities Superficial thrombophlebitis	None	None
Low risk		
Previous VTE related to trauma or major surgery in patient without underlying thrombophilia	Prophylactic doses of heparin vs. no therapy	Prophylactic doses of heparin vs. no therapy
Moderate risk		
Idiopathic thrombosis VTE in prior pregnancy Underlying thrombophilia but *NOT* • homozygous factor V Leiden • heterozygous factor V Leiden and prothrombin G20210A or AT-III deficiency	Heparin or LMWH in prophylactic doses administered subcutaneously in divided doses	Heparin or LMWH in prophylactic doses administered subcutaneously in divided doses
High risk		
Life-threatening thrombosis Recent thrombosis Recurrent thrombosis Chronic anticoagulation APS with prior thrombosis or stroke Underlying thrombophilia • AT-III decifiency • homozygous factor V Leiden • homozygous prothrombin G20210A • heterozygous factor V Leiden and prothrombin G20210A or AT-III deficiency	Heparin in adjusted-dose prophylaxis or twice daily low molecular weight heparin	Initially heparin and warfarin for at least 5 days then warfarin administered daily in doses to maintain international normalized ratio >3.0 for at least 6 weeks

Low molecular weight heparin (LMWH) may be used in pregnancy but there is a lack of data regarding adequate dosing so antifactor Xa levels may be monitored. Epidural anesthesia should be withheld until 24 hours after the last injection of LMWH.

Unfractionated Heparin	
Low dose prophylaxis	**Adjusted dose prophylaxis**
5,000-7,500 U every 12 hours during the first trimester 7,500-10,000 U every 12 hours during the second trimester 10,000 U every 12 hours during the third trimester unless the APTT is elevated. The APTT may be checked near term and the heparin dose reduced if prolonged. *OR* 5,000-10,000 U every 12 hours during the entire pregnancy	≥ 10,000 U twice to three times daily to achieve APTT of 1.5-2.5

Low Molecular Weight Heparin	
Low dose prophylaxis	**Adjusted dose prophylaxis**
Dalteparin 5,000 U once or twice daily Enoxaparin 40 mg once or twice daily	Dalteparin 5,000-10,000 U every 12 hours Enoxapin 30-80 mg every 12 hours

Source: American College of Obstetricians and Gynecologists: *Thromboembolism in Pregnancy*. ACOG Practice Bulletin #19, August 2000. ACOG, Washington, DC © 2000. Reproduced with the permission of the publisher.

THROMBOCYTOPENIA IN PREGNANCY
Fast Facts
• defined as platelet count < 150,000/μl,
    • repeat platelet count and obtain a CBC to exclude pancytopenia and lab artifact
• occurs in 8% of pregnancies
• obtaining antiplatelet antibodies is not recommended (does not help with the Dx or Rx)
• epidural anesthesia should not be given if maternal platelets are < 50k

Gestational Thrombocytopenia
• most common cause of thrombocytopenia in pregnancy (2/3 of cases)
• manifests itself usually in the third trimester and is usually mild (rarely <70k)
• usually not associated with fetal thrombocytopenia thus no risk for fetal hemorrhage
• does not require any other testing than routine antepartum platelet count every 1-2 months
• can be difficult to distinguish from ITP since antibodies can also be present.
    • usually milder, occurs later in gestation and no maternal history of thrombocytopenia

Neonatal Alloimmune Thrombocytopenia
• occurs in 1:1000 pregnancies
• caused by maternal antibodies to paternal originating platelet antigens (HPA-1 and -2)
• similar to Rh disease but can occur during a first pregnancy
• maternal platelet count is usually normal
• 10-20% of neonates will develop intracranial hemorrhage which often occurs *in utero*
• treatment is IVIG (+/- steroids, fetal transfusion) to increase fetal platelet count
• assessment of fetal platelet count prior to treatment is controversial
    • fetal blood sampling at 22-24 weeks gestation may optimize medical treatment
• most investigators suggest delivery at 37 wks
    • sample fetal platelet count to determine mode of delivery (<50k consider cesarean)
• recurrence rate is extremely high consider testing parents for platelet incompatabilty

Immune Thrombocytopenia Purpura (ITP)
• occurs in 1:1000 to 1:10,000 pregnancies
• caused by maternal IgG antiplatelet antibodies destroying maternal and fetal platelets
• maternal platelet count usually < 100k, maternal count correlates poorly with fetal count
• 15% of infants to mothers with ITP will have counts < 50k, 5% with counts < 20k
• rate of intracranial hemorrhage is extremely low (< 1%) as compared to neonatal alloimmune TC
• maternal treatment for fetal indications is not recommended.
• obtain platelet counts frequently
    • maternal therapy indicated for platelet count < 50K
        • prednisone 1-2mg/kg/d, prn IVIG and platelet transfusion
• obtaining fetal platelet count is probably not warranted
    • mode of delivery should be based upon obstetric considerations only
        • Cesarean section does not seem to decrease risk of intracranial hemorrhage

Pregnancy-induced Hypertension (PIH)
• etiology in 20% of cases
• cause is unknown but platelet count rarely less than 20k
• primary treatment in the setting of PIH or HELLP syndrome is delivery
• consider increasing the platelet count to > 50k if considering cesarean section and/or epidural
• consider immediate postpartum uterine curettage for faster recovery

OBSTETRICS

α AND β THALASSEMIA

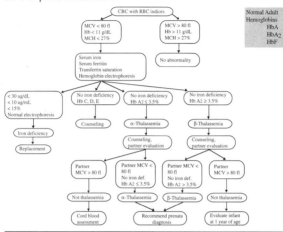

Normal Adult Hemoglobins	
HbA	2α, 2β
HbA₂	2α, 2δ
HbF	2α, 2γ

	Deletions	Globulin	Clinical Effects
α-Thalassemia			
α-Thalassemia trait	2 genes	50%	Mild anemia, microcytosis, hypochromia
Hb H disease	3 genes	25%	Moderate anemia, transfusion rarely, splenectomy occasionally
Bart Hb	4 genes	None	Severe intrauterine anemia, hydrops
β-Thalassemia			
β-Thalassemia trait	Point mutations	50%	Mild anemia, microcytosis, hypochromia
β-Thalassemia intermediate	Point mutations	25%	Moderate anemia, transfusion occ, hepatosplenomegaly, bone deformities, iron overload
β-Thalassemia major	Point mutations	None	Severe anemia, chronic transfusion, hepatosplenomegaly, bone deformities, iron overload

From American College of Obstetricians and Gynecologists: *Hemoglobinopathies in pregnancy*. Technical Bulletin 185. ACOG, Washington, DC © 1993. Reproduced with permission of the publisher.

OBSTETRICS

GUIDELINES FOR DIAGNOSTIC IMAGING IN PREGNANCY
Fast Facts
• diagnostic X-ray is a frequent source of patient anxiety
• no single diagnostic X-ray procedure is enough to threaten the well-being of the embryo or fetus
• risk of fetal anomalies, growth restriction or spontaneous abortion not increased at exposure level of < 5 rad
• threshold for mental retardation probably 20-40 rad

Procedure	Fetal Exposure
Chest X-ray (2 views)	0.02-0.07 mrad
Abdominal film (single only)	100 mrad
Intravenous pyelogram	> 1 rad*
Hip film (single view)	200 mrad
Mammography	7-20 mrad
Barium enema or small bowel series	2-4 rad
CT scan of head or chest	< 1 rad
CT scan of abdomen and lumbar spine	3.5 rad
CT pelvimetry	250 mrad

* Exposure depends on number of films

Source: American College of Obstetricians and Gynecologists. *Guidelines for diagnostic imaging during pregnancy.* Committee Opinion 158, 1995:1-4.

Guidelines from ACOG
1) X-ray exposure from a single diagnostic procedure does not result in harmful fetal effects
   • exposure to < 5 rad not associated with adverse outcome
2) Concern about possible fetal effects should not prevent indicated diagnostic testing but consider use of nonionizing radiation when possible
3) MRI and ultrasound are safe but safety of MRI in the first trimester is less well studied
4) Use of radioactive isotopes of iodine is contraindicated

OBSTETRICS

HEPATITIS

Viral Agent	Virion Structure	Genome size and nature	Incubation period	Clinical severity	Transmission	Prevention
Hepatitis A	28 nm No envelope	7.5 kb RNA ss, pos	15-60 days	Mild	Fecal/oral from food and water Parenteral relatively rare	Immunization Sanitation with clean water and separate waste disposal Hand washing Cooking food Peeling fruits and vegetables
Hepatitis B	42 nm Enveloped	3.2 kb DNA Partial ds	45-160 days	Occasionally severe	Parenteral and IV drug use Sexual contact Perinatal Transfusion-associated (rare)	Immunization Protection against exposure to bodily fluids (including blood) Safe sexual practices Universal precautions by healthcare workers
Hepatitis C	38-50 nm Enveloped	9.4 kb RNA ss, pos	14-180 days	Mild	Parenteral and IV drug use Sexual contact Perinatal Transfusion-associated (rare)	Similar to hepatitis B No vaccine available Universal precautions
Hepatitis D	43 nm Enveloped	1.7 kb RNA ss, neg	42-180 days Depends on superinfection vs. co-infection	Occasionally severe	Parenteral Sexual contact Perinatal	Sterilization and disinfection of medical equipment and environmental surfaces Hepatitis B vaccine Universal precautions
Hepatitis E	32 nm No envelope	7.8 kb RNA ss, pos	15-60 days	Mild	Drinking water in endemic areas Person-to-person transmission appears low	Personal hygiene Boil drinking water Avoid uncooked food

Source: Modified from Younossi ZM. Viral hepatitis guide for practicing physicians. *Cleveland Clinic J Med.* 2000;67 Suppl:6-23. Reproduced with permission.

HEPATITIS B

	Incubation	Late Incubation / Early Acute	Early Acute	Acute	Acute but seroconversion in progress	Convalescent Window	Early Recovery	Recovery
HBeAg			|	|				
HBsAg		|	|	|	|			
Anti-HBc IgM				|	|			
Anti-HBc				|	|	|	|	|
Anti-HBe					|	|	|	|
Anti-HBs							|	|
Duration	4-12 w	1-2 w	2 weeks - 3 months			3-6 months	Years	
Infectivity	Infectious					Potentially Infectious	Immune	

Curve labels: HBsAg, HBeAg, Anti-HBcIgM, Anti-HBc, Anti-HBe, Anti-HBs

83

OBSTETRICS

HEPATITIS C
Fast Facts
• hepatitis C is now the leading indication for liver transplantation in many US medical centers
• approximately 50% of hepatitis C cases result from IV drug use
• risk of sexual transmission in a discordant monogamous couple is 5% over 10-20 years
• 85-90% of infected patients are unable to clear the virus and are chronically infected
• no guidelines for hepatitis C and pregnancy exist
    • perinatal transmission probably 5-6% of cases but higher in HIV-positive women
    • breast feeding is not an established risk factor
    • pregnant women cannot be treated with alpha interferon or ribavirin

Screening and Evaluation

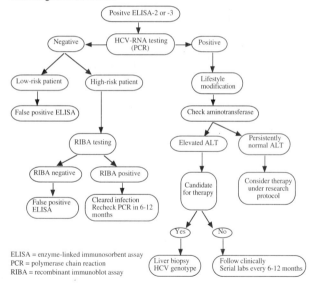

ELISA = enzyme-linked immunosorbent assay
PCR = polymerase chain reaction
RIBA = recombinant immunoblot assay

Source: Sarbah SA, Younossi ZM. Hepatitis C: an update on the silent epidemic. *J Clin Gastroenterol*. 2000;30(2):125-143.

MANAGEMENT OF TUBERCULOSIS IN PREGNANCY

Fast Facts
• total number of cases of TB in 1999 (17,500)
• pregnancy has no effect on tuberculin sensitivity

Mantoux Test
• 0.1 mL of PPD tuberculin (5 Tuberculin Units)
• place intradermal
• read after 48-72 hours
• positive test

5 mm
• close contact with infectious TB patients
• CXR containing old fibrotic lesion
• known or suspected HIV infection

15 mm
• positive in all other persons

10 mm
• HIV infection
• silicosis
• abnormal CXR
• prolonged corticosteroid therapy
• diabetes mellitus
• hematologic, renal, cardiac disease
• member of an ethnic or socioeconomic group with high prevalence
• IV drug user
• resident of a long-term care facility

BCG (Bacillus of Calmette and Guerin)
• vaccination used in many foreign countries to control TB
• PPD sensitivity after BCG is variable
• positive tuberculin test should be evaluated as for other patients

Evaluation

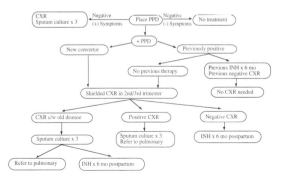

From Stanford Clinic Pulmonary Tuberculosis Exposure Control Plan, July 1994.

OBSTETRICS

HUMAN IMMUNODEFICIENCY VIRUS (HIV)
Fast Facts
- perinatal transmission of HIV accounts for most infections in children
- risk of perinatal transmission is about 25%

Risk Factor	Possible Preventative Intervention
Antepartum risk factors	
Advanced HIV disease • low CD4 count • high plasma viral load	Antiretroviral therapy
Intrapartum risk factors	
Prolonged rupture of membranes	Scheduled C/S, avoiding artificial rupture of membranes
Vaginal delivery	Scheduled C/S
Increased exposure to maternal blood	Scheduled C/S, avoiding fetal scalp electrodes, scalp sampling and episiotomy
Postpartum risk factors	
Breastfeeding	Avoiding breastfeeding

Prenatal Care
- monitor CD4 counts and viral load during each trimester if possible
- check CD4 counts to determine need for *Pneumocystis carinii* prophylaxis
  - initiate prophylaxis when CD4 <200/mm^3
    - trimethoprim/sulfamethoxazole (Septra DS) 800 mg/160 mg q day
    - IV pentamidine for severe disease in patients intolerant of TMP-SMX
- check for tuberculosis with two tests for anergy as well

Laboratory Evaluation
Routine prenatal labs
Blood type and screen Rubella titer CBC Urine culture Hepatitis B surface antigen RPR or VDRL for syphilis
Immune status
CD4 count Quantitative plasma viral load
Infections
Gonorrhea and chlamydia testing Hepatitis C antibody PPD for tuberculosis Toxoplasmosis antibody (IgG and IgM) Cytomegalovirus antibody (IgG and IgM)

AIDS Clinical Trial Group Protocol 076
Antepartum
Initiate zidovudine (ZDV) at 14-34 weeks' gestation; continue throughout pregnancy a) ZDV 100 mg PO 5 times a day (q 4 h while awake) b) Alternatives: ZDV 200 mg PO q8h ZDV 300 mg PO q12h
Intrapartum
ZDV 2 mg/kg IV over 1 hour, followed by continuous infusion of 1 mg/kg IV until delivery
Postpartum
Neonatal treatment with PO ZDV syrup 2 mg/kg every 6 hours for the first 6 weeks of life, beginning 8-12 hours following birth

Source: Dinsmoor MJ. Managing the HIV-infected pregnant patient. *Cont OB/GYN*, December 2000. Reproduced with permission of Medical Economics Publishing, Montvale, NJ.

HUMAN IMMUNODEFICIENCY VIRUS (HIV)

Medication	Drug regimen	Comparison group	Transmission rate	Reference
Zidovudine	Given antepartum, intrapartum and postpartum	Placebo	Reduced mother-to-child transmission rate by 66% (from 22.6% to 7.6%)	Connor et al, *NEJM* 1994;331:1173-1180.
Zidovudine	Given antepartum from week 36 and intrapartum	Placebo	Reduced transmission by 50% (from 19% to 9%)	Shaffer et al, *Lancet* 1999; 353:773-780.
Zidovudine and lamivudine	Given intrapartum and postpartum for 1 week for mother and neonate	Placebo	Reduced transmission by 38% (from 17% to 10%)	Saba et al, Sixth Conference on Retroviruses, Chicago, IL, January 1999, Abstract S-7.
Nevirapine	200 mg at onset of labor, one dose to neonate	Zidovudine intrapartum and to neonate	Reduced transmission by 50% (25% to 13%)	Guay et al, *Lancet* 1999; 354:795-802.

Currently Available Antiretroviral Agents

Nucleoside reverse transcriptase inhibitors (NRTI)

Generic name	Trade name	FDA pregnancy category
Abacavir	Ziagen	C
Didanosine (ddI)	Videx	B
Lamivudine (3TC)	Epivir	C
Lamivudine + zidovudine	Combivir	C
Stavudine (d4T)	Zerit	C
Zalcitabine	Hivid	C
Zidovudine (ZDV, AZT)	Retrovir	C

Nonnucleoside reverse transcriptase inhibitors (NNRTI)

Generic name	Trade name	FDA pregnancy category
Delavirdine	Rescriptor	C
Efavirenz	Sustiva*	C
Nevirapine	Viramune	C

Protease inhibitors (PI)

Generic name	Trade name	FDA pregnancy category
Amprenavir	Agenerase*	C
Indinavir	Crixivan	C
Nelfinavir	Viracept	B
Ritonavir	Norvir	B
Saquinavir	Fortovase (soft gel capsule) Invirase (hard gel capsule)	B

* currently considered contraindicated in pregnancy

Source: Dinsmoor MJ. Managing the HIV-infected pregnant patient. *Cont OB/GYN*, December 2000. Reproduced with permission of Medical Economics Publishing, Montvale, NJ.

OBSTETRICS

HERPES SIMPLEX VIRUS
Fast Facts
• positive cultures have been reported in 0.2-7.4% of pregnancies
• maternal antibodies appear 7 days after primary infection
    • peak levels in 2-3 weeks
    • remain positive for life
• HSV shedding occurs at time of delivery in 0.1-0.4% of all patients

Neonatal Infection
• rate of infection is approximately 0.01-0.04% of all deliveries
    • 10% reduction over HSV shedding likely result of maternal antibodies conferring protective effect
• 70% of neonatal infections occur in women with no history of HSV
• infection may occur with either HSV-1 (25%) or HSV-2 (75%)
• mechanism of infection
    • passage through infected birth canal
    • ascending infection (especially with ruptured membranes)
    • close contact with infected mother or relative
    • close contact with infected health care provider
• rate of infection dependent on primary vs. recurrent HSV
    • primary maternal infection at time of vaginal delivery
        • 50% neonatal infection rate
    • recurrent maternal infection at time of vaginal delivery
        • 4% neonatal infection rate
• 60% of infants with neonatal HSV from mother with primary HSV will die
    • 50% of survivors will have serious sequelae

Antepartum Management
• culture should be done only to confirm diagnosis with visible lesions
• weekly HSV cultures in asymptomatic mothers not necessary
• amniocentesis to rule out intrauterine infection not recommended

Management Recommendations
The following are based on Level B scientific evidence:
• Women with primary HSV during pregnancy should be treated with antiviral therapy.
• Cesarean delivery should be performed on women with first-episode HSV who have active genital lesions at delivery.
• For women at or beyond 36 weeks with a first episode HSV occuring during the current pregnancy, antiviral therapy should be considered.

The following are based on Level C information:
• Cesarean delivery should be performed on women with recurrent HSV infection who have active genital lesions or prodromal symptoms at delivery.
• Expectant management of patients with preterm labor or preterm PROM and HSV may be warranted.
• For women at or beyond 36 weeks and who are at risk for recurrent HSV, antiviral therapy may be considered.
Cesarean delivery should not be performed on women without active lesions or prodromal symptoms during labor.

Source: American College of Obstetricians and Gynecologists. *Management of Herpes in Pregnancy.* ACOG Practice Bulletin #8, October 1999.

VARICELLA
Fast Facts
- 1/10,000 pregnancies complicated by maternal chickenpox
- 25% of maternal infections result in evidence of fetal infection
- 1st trimester maternal varicella results in <2.5-3% risk of congenital varicella syndrome (skin scarring, limb hypoplasia, CNS, eye abnormalities)
- avoid delivery if possible during 7 day window
    - 2 days before onset of maternal rash, 5 days after onset of rash
    - 11-21 days between exposure and rash (mean 15 days)
- IV acyclovir can be used for severe maternal infections
    - 10-30% of pregnant varicella patients develop varicella pneumonia
        - 40% mortality rate
- no fetal risk in cases of maternal herpes zoster (shingles)
- immunize if non-immune preconception or postpartum

Management

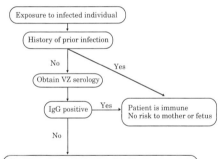

OBSTETRICS

RUBELLA

Fast Facts

- infection can be communicated 7 days before and 4 days after appearance of rash
- rash occurs 2-3 weeks following exposure
  - usually lasts 3 days "3 day measles"
- rate of fetal infection depends on stage of gestation
  - <11 weeks → 90% risk of congenital infection
  - 11-12 wks → 33%
  - 13-14 wks → 11%
  - 15-16 wks → 24%
  - > 16 weeks → 0%
- risk of fetal anomalies also dependent on gestational age
  - 1st trimester → 25%
    - 1st month → 50%
    - 2nd month → 25%
    - 3rd month → 10%
  - 2nd trimester → <1%
    - 16-20 weeks: sensory only
  - >20 weeks: no reported cases

Management

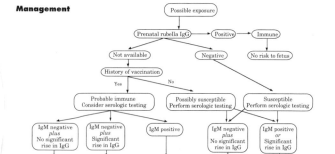

Post-exposure testing
   IgM and IgG drawn ASAP and paired IgG ASAP and in 4-5 weeks

Post-rash testing
   IgM and IgG drawn ASAP after rash and paired IgG ASAP after the rash and in 2-3 weeks

Source: American College of Obstetricians and Gynecologists: *Rubella and Pregnancy*. Technical Bulletin 171. ACOG, Washington, DC © 1992. Reproduced with permission of the publisher, the American College of Obstetricians and Gynecologists.

TOXOPLASMOSIS

Fast Facts

• 1/3 of women have been exposed through ingestion of undercooked meat and contact with cat feces
• presence of IgG indicates immunity, IgM appears within 1 week and lasts for months
• increasing gestational age increases infection rate but diminishes severity
• rate of fetal infection
    • 1st trimester: 15%
    • 2nd trimester: 30%
    • 3rd trimester: 60%
• fetal malformations
    • IUGR, microcephaly, chorioretinitis, intracranial calcifications

Management

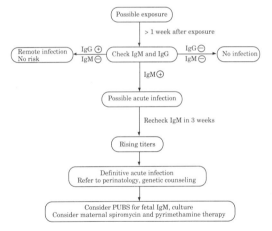

Possible exposure

> 1 week after exposure

Remote infection
No risk

IgG ⊕
IgM ⊖

Check IgM and IgG

IgG ⊖
IgM ⊖

No infection

IgM ⊕

Possible acute infection

Recheck IgM in 3 weeks

Rising titers

Definitive acute infection
Refer to perinatology, genetic counseling

Consider PUBS for fetal IgM, culture
Consider maternal spiromycin and pyrimethamine therapy

OBSTETRICS

CYTOMEGALOVIRUS (CMV)

Fast Facts
- complicates 0.2-2% of pregnancies
- usually asymptomatic
- 80% of mothers have been already infected
- risk of malformations decrease with gestational age
- CMV tetrad: mental retardation, microcephaly, chorioretinitis, cerebral calcifications

Consequences of CMV in Pregnancy

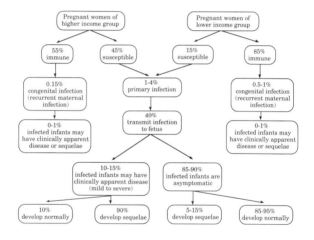

Source: Stagno S and Whitley RJ. Herpesvirus infections of pregnancy, Part I: Cytomegalovirus and Epstein-Barr virus infections. *NEJM* 1985; 313(20):1270-4. Reproduced with permission of the publisher.

VACCINES AND PREGNANCY

Viral Agent	Risk from disease to pregnant woman	Risk from disease to fetus or neonate	Type of immunizing agent	Risk from immunizing agent to fetus	Indications for immunization during pregnancy	Dose schedule	Comments
LIVE VIRUS VACCINES							
Measles	Significant morbidity, low mortality; not altered by pregnancy	Significant increase in abortion rate; may cause fetal malformations	Live attenuated virus vaccine	None confirmed	Contraindicated (see immune globulins)	Single dose SC, preferably as measles-mumps-rubella (MMR)	Vaccination of susceptible women should be part of postpartum care
Mumps	Low morbidity and mortality; not altered by pregnancy	Probable increased rate of abortion in first trimester	Live attenuated virus vaccine	None confirmed	Contraindicated	Single dose SC, preferably as measles-mumps-rubella (MMR)	Vaccination of susceptible women should be part of postpartum care
Poliomyelitis	No increased incidence in pregnancy, but may be more severe if it does occur	Anoxic fetal damage reported; 50% mortality in neonatal cases	Live attenuated virus (oral polio vaccine (OPV)) and enhanced-potency inactivated virus (e-IPV) vaccine	None confirmed	Not routinely recommended for women in U.S., except persons at increased risk of exposure	Primary 2 doses of e-IPV SC at 4-8 week intervals and a 3rd dose 6-12 months after the second dose. Immediate protection: 1 dose OPV orally (in outbreak setting)	Vaccine indicated for susceptible pregnant women travelling in endemic areas or in other high-risk situations
Rubella	Low morbidity and mortality; not altered by pregnancy	High rate of abortion and congenital rubella syndrome	Live attenuated virus vaccine	None confirmed	Contraindicated	Single dose SC, preferably as measles-mumps-rubella (MMR)	Teratogenicity of vaccine is theoretic; not confirmed to date; vaccination of susceptible women should be part of postpartum care
Yellow fever	Significant morbidity and mortality; not altered by pregnancy	Unknown	Live attenuated virus vaccine	Unknown	Contraindicated except if exposure is unavoidable	Single dose SC	Postponement of travel preferable to vaccination, if pregnancy possible

Source: American College of Obstetricians and Gynecologists, *Immunization During Pregnancy*, ACOG Technical Bulletin, Number 160. October 1991. Copyright 1991 American College of Obstetricians and Gynecologists. Reproduced with permission.

OBSTETRICS

VACCINES AND PREGNANCY

Viral Agent	Risk from disease to pregnant woman	Risk from disease to fetus or neonate	Type of immunizing agent	Risk from immunizing agent to fetus	Indications for immunization during pregnancy	Dose schedule	Comments
INACTIVATED VIRUS VACCINES							
Influenza	Possible increase in morbidity and mortality during epidemic of new antigenic strain	Possible increased abortion rate; no malformations confirmed	Inactivated virus vaccine	None confirmed	Women with serious underlying diseases; public health authorities to be consulted for current recommendations	One dose IM every year	
Rabies	Near 100% fatality; not altered by pregnancy	Determined by maternal disease	Killed virus vaccine	Unknown	Indications for prophylaxis not altered by pregnancy; each case considered individually	Public health authorities to be consulted for indications, dosage and route of administration	
Hepatitis B	Possible increased severity during third trimester	Possible increase in abortion rate and prematurity; neonatal hepatitis can occur; high risk of newborn carrier state	Recombinant vaccine	None reported	Pre- and post-exposure for women at risk of infection	Three- or four-dose series	Used with hepatitis B immune globulin for some exposures; exposed newborn needs vaccination as soon as possible

Source: American College of Obstetricians and Gynecologists. *Immunization During Pregnancy*. ACOG Technical Bulletin, Number 160, October 1991. Copyright 1991 American College of Obstetricians and Gynecologists. Reproduced with permission.

VACCINES AND PREGNANCY

Viral Agent	Risk from disease to pregnant woman	Risk from disease to fetus or neonate	Type of immunizing agent	Risk from immunizing agent to fetus	Indications for immunization during pregnancy	Dose schedule	Comments
INACTIVATED BACTERIAL VACCINES							
Cholera	Significant morbidity and mortality; more severe during third trimester	Increased risk of fetal death during third-trimester maternal illness	Killed bacterial vaccine	None confirmed	Indications not altered by pregnancy; vaccination recommended only in unusual outbreak situations	Single dose SC or IM depending on manufacturer's recommendations when indicated	
Plague	Significant morbidity and mortality; not altered by pregnancy	Determined by maternal disease	Killed bacterial vaccine	None reported	Selective vaccination of exposed persons	Public health authorities to be consulted for indications, dosage and route of administration	
Pneumococcus	No increased risk during pregnancy and no increase in severity of disease	Unknown	Polyvalent polysaccharide vaccine	No data available on use during pregnancy	Indications not altered by pregnancy; vaccine used only for high-risk individuals	In adults, 1 SC or IM dose only; consider repeat dose in 6 years for high-risk individuals	
Typhoid	Significant morbidity and mortality; not altered by pregnancy	Unknown	Killed or live attenuated oral bacterial vaccine	None confirmed	Not recommended routinely except for close, continued exposure or travel to endemic areas	**Killed:** *Primary:* 2 injections SC at least 4 weeks apart. *Booster:* Single dose SC or ID (depending on type of product used) every 3 years. **Oral:** *Primary:* 4 doses on alternative days. *Booster:* Schedule not yet determined	

From American College of Obstetricians and Gynecologists. *Immunization During Pregnancy.* ACOG Technical Bulletin, Number 160, October 1991. Copyright 1991 American College of Obstetricians and Gynecologists. Reproduced with permission.

VACCINES AND PREGNANCY

Viral Agent	Risk from disease to pregnant woman	Risk from disease to fetus or neonate	Type of immunizing agent	Risk from immunizing agent to fetus	Indications for immunization during pregnancy	Dose schedule	Comments
SPECIFIC IMMUNE GLOBULINS							
Hepatitis B	Possible increased severity during third trimester	Possible increase in abortion rate and prematurity; neonatal hepatitis can occur; high risk of carriage in newborn	Hepatitis B immune globulin	None reported	Postexposure prophylaxis	Depends on exposure; consult Immunization Practices Advisory Committee recommendations (IM)	Usually given with HBV vaccine; exposed newborn needs immediate postexposure prophylaxis
Rabies	Near 100% fatality; not altered by pregnancy	Determined by maternal disease	Rabies immune globulin	None reported	Postexposure prophylaxis	Half dose at injury site, half dose in deltoid	Used in conjunction with rabies killed virus vaccine
Tetanus	Severe morbidity; mortality 21%	Neonatal tetanus mortality 60%	Tetanus immune globulin	None reported	Postexposure prophylaxis	One dose IM	Used in conjunction with tetanus toxoid
Varicella	Possible increase in severe varicella pneumonia	Can cause congenital varicella with increased mortality in neonatal period; very rarely causes congenital defects	Varicella-zoster immune globulin (obtained from American Red Cross)	None reported	Can be considered for healthy pregnant women exposed to varicella to protect against maternal, not congenital, infection	One dose IM within 96 hours of exposure	Indicated also for newborns of mothers who developed varicella within 4 days prior to delivery or 2 days following delivery; approximately 90-95% of adults are immune to varicella; not indicated for prevention of congenital varicella

Source: American College of Obstetricians and Gynecologists. *Immunization During Pregnancy*. ACOG Technical Bulletin, Number 160, October 1991. Copyright 1991 American College of Obstetricians and Gynecologists. Reproduced with permission.

VACCINES AND PREGNANCY

Viral Agent	Risk from disease to pregnant woman	Risk from disease to fetus or neonate	Type of immunizing agent	Risk from immunizing agent to fetus	Indications for immunization during pregnancy	Dose schedule	Comments
TOXOIDS							
Tetanus-diphtheria	Severe morbidity; tetanus mortality ~30%; diphtheria mortality 10%; unaltered by pregnancy	Neonatal tetanus mortality 60%	Combined tetanus-diphtheria toxoids preferred; adult tetanus-diphtheria formulation	None confirmed	Lack of primary series, or no booster within past 10 years	Primary: 2 doses IM at 1-2 month interval with a 3rd dose 6-12 months after the 2nd. Booster: Single dose IM every 10 years, after completion of primary series	Updating of immune status should be part of antepartum care
STANDARD IMMUNE GLOBULINS							
Hepatitis A	Possible increased severity during third trimester	Probable increase in abortion rate and prematurity; possible transmission to neonate at delivery if mother is incubating the virus or is acutely ill at that time	Standard immune globulin	None reported	Postexposure prophylaxis	0.02 mL/kg IM in one dose of immune globulin	Immune globulin should be given as soon as possible and within 2 weeks of exposure; infants born to mothers who are incubating the virus or are acutely ill at delivery should receive one dose of 0.5 mL as soon as possible after birth
Measles	Significant morbidity, low mortality, not altered by pregnancy	Significant increase in abortion rate; may cause malformations	Standard immune globulin	None reported	Postexposure prophylaxis	0.25 mL/kg IM in one dose of immune globulin up to 15 mL	Unclear if it prevents abortion; must be given within 6 days of exposure

Source: American College of Obstetricians and Gynecologists. *Immunization During Pregnancy.* ACOG Technical Bulletin, Number 160, October 1991. Copyright 1991 American College of Obstetricians and Gynecologists. Reproduced with permission.

OBSTETRICS

TERATOLOGY
Agents Not Documented as Teratogens.
*Paternal exposure to any agent has not been shown to be teratogenic.

Drugs and chemicals
Acetaminophen
Acyclovir
Antiemetics
(e.g., phenothiazines, trimethobenzamide)
Antihistamines
(e.g., doxylamine)
Aspartame
Aspirin
Caffeine
Hair spray
Marijuana
Metronidazole
Minor tranquilizers
(e.g., meprobamate, chlordiazepoxide, fluoxetine)
Occupational chemical agents

Oral contraceptives
Pesticides
Trimethoprim-sulfamethoxazole
Vaginal spermicides
Zidovudine

Infections
Herpes simplex type 2 virus
Parvovirus B19

Electromagnetic fields from video display
terminals
Heat

Sources of Current Teratogen Information

Eastern United States
Massachusetts Teratogen Information Service
Boston, Massachusetts
(617) 466-8474

Western United States
Pregnancy Riskline
Salt Lake City, Utah
(801) 328-2229

Micromedex, Inc.
REPRORISK (REPROTEXT, REPROTOX, Shepard's
Catalog of Teratogenic Agents and TERIS)
Englewood, CO
(800) 525-9083

Teratogen Information System
TERIS and Shepard's Catalog of Teratogenic Agents
Seattle, WA
(206) 543-2465

National Library of Medicine,
MEDLARS Service Desk
GRATEFUL MED
(TOXLINE, TOXNET and MEDLINE)
Bethesda, MD
(800) 638-8480

Reproductive Toxicology Center
REPROTOX
Columbia Hospital for Women
Washington, DC
(202) 293-5137

Shepard's Catalog of Teratogenic Agents
University of Washington
Seattle, WA
(206) 543-3373

Source: American College of Obstetricians and Gynecologists. *Teratology.* ACOG Educational Bulletin, Number 236, April 1997. Copyright 1997 American College of Obstetricians and Gynecologists. Reproduced with permission.

TERATOLOGY

Agent	Effects	Comments
Alcohol	Growth restriction before and after birth, mental retardation, microcephaly, midfacial hypoplasia producing atypical facial appearance, renal and cardiac defects, various other major and minor malformations.	Nutritional deficiency, smoking, and multiple drug use confounded data. Risk due to ingestion of up to one to two drinks per day is not well defined but may cause a small reduction in average birth weight. Fetuses of women who ingest six drinks per day are at a 40% risk of developing some features of the fetal alcohol syndrome.
Androgens and testosterone derivatives (e.g., danazol)	Virilization of female, advanced genital development in males.	Effects are dose-dependent and related to the stage of embryonic development at the time of exposure. Given before 9 weeks of gestation, labioscrotal fusion can be produced; clitoromegaly can occur with exposure at any gestational age. Risk related to incidental brief androgenic exposure is minimal
Angiotensin-converting enzyme (ACE) inhibitors (e.g., enalapril, captopril)	Fetal renal tubular dysplasia, oligohydramnios, neonatal renal failure, lack of cranial ossification, intrauterine growth restriction.	Incidence of fetal morbidity is 30%. The risk increases with second- and third-trimester use, leading to in utero fetal hypertension, decreased renal blood flow, and renal failure.
Coumarin derivatives (e.g., warfarin)	Nasal hypoplasia and stippled bone epiphyses are most common; other effects include broad short hands with shortened phalanges, ophthalmologic abnormalities, intrauterine growth restriction, developmental delay, anomalies of neck and central nervous system.	Risk to a seriously affected child is considered to be 15-25% when anticoagulants that inhibit vitamin K are used in the first trimester, especially during 6-9 weeks of gestation. Later drug exposure may be associated with spontaneous abortion, stillbirth, central nervous system abnormalities, abruptio placentae, and fetal or neonatal hemorrhage.
Carbamazepine	Neural tube defects, minor craniofacial defects, fingernail hypoplasia, microcephaly, developmental delay, intrauterine growth restriction.	Risk of neural tube defects, mostly lumbosacral, is 1-2% when used alone during first trimester and increased when used with other antiepileptic agents.
Folic acid antagonists (methotrexate and aminopterin)	Increased risk for spontaneous abortions, various anomalies.	These drugs are contraindicated for the treatment of psoriasis in pregnancy and must be used with extreme caution in the treatment of malignancy. Cytotoxic drugs are potentially teratogenic. Effects of aminopterin are well documented. Folic acid antagonists used during the first trimester produce a malformation rate of up to 30% in fetuses that survive.
Cocaine	Bowel atresias; congenital malformations of the heart, limbs, face and genitourinary tract; microcephaly; intrauterine growth restriction, cerebral infarctions.	Risks may be affected by other factors and concurrent abuse of multiple substances. Maternal and pregnancy complications include sudden death and placental abruption.
Diethylstilbestrol	Clear-cell adenocarcinoma of the vagina or cervix, vaginal adenosis, abnormalities of cervix and uterus, abnormalities of the testes, possible infertility in males and females.	Vaginal adenosis is detected in more than 50% of women whose mothers took these drugs before 9 weeks of gestation. Risk for vaginal adenocarcinoma is low. Males exposed in utero may have a 25% incidence of epididymal cysts, hypotrophic testes, abnormal spermatozoa, and induration of the testes.
Lead	Increased abortion rate, stillbirths.	Fetal central nervous system development may be adversely affected by determining preconceptional lead levels for those at risk may be useful.
Lithium	Congenital heart disease, in particular, Ebstein anomaly.	Risk of heart malformations due to first-trimester exposure is low. The effect is not as significant as reported in earlier studies. Exposure in the last month of gestation may produce toxic effects on the thyroid, kidneys, and neuromuscular systems.

OBSTETRICS

TERATOLOGY

Agent	Effects	Comments
Organic mercury	Cerebral atrophy, microcephaly, mental retardation, spasticity, seizures, blindness.	Cerebral palsy can occur even when exposure is in the third trimester. Exposed individuals include consumers of fish and grain contaminated with methyl mercury.
Phenytoin	Intrauterine growth restriction, mental retardation, microcephaly, dysmorphic craniofacial features, cardiac defect, hypoplastic nails and distal phalanges.	The full syndrome is seen in less than 10% of children exposed in utero, but up to 30% have some manifestations. Mild to moderate mental retardation is found in some children who have severe physical stigmata. The effect may depend on whether the fetus inherits a mutant gene that decreases production of epoxide hydrolase, an enzyme necessary to decrease the teratogen phenytoin epoxide.
Streptomycin and kanamycin	Hearing loss, eighth-nerve damage.	No ototoxicity in the fetus has been reported from use of gentamicin or vancomycin.
Tetracycline	Hypoplasia of tooth enamel, incorporation of tetracycline into bone and teeth, permanent yellow- brown discoloration of deciduous teeth.	Drug has no known effect unless exposure occurs in second or third trimester.
Thalidomide	Bilateral limb deficiencies, anotia and microtia, cardiac and gastrointestinal anomalies.	Of children whose mothers used thalidomide between 35 and 50 days of gestation, 20% show the effect.
Trimethadione and paramethadione	Clef lip or cleft palate, cardiac defects, growth deficiency, microcephaly, mental retardation, characteristic facial appearance, ophthalmologic, limb, and genitourinary tract abnormalities.	Risk for defects or spontaneous abortion is 60-80% with first-trimester exposure. A syndrome including V-shaped eyebrows, low-set ears, high arched palate, and irregular dentition has been identified. These drugs are no longer used during pregnancy due to the availability of more effective, less toxic agents.
Valproic acid	Neural tube defects, especially spine bifida, minor facial defects.	Exposure must occur prior to normal closure of neural tube during first trimester to produce open defect (incidence of approximately 1%).
Vitamin A and its derivatives (e.g., Isotretinoin, etretinate and retinoids)	Increased abortion rate, microtia, central nervous system defects, thymic agenesis, cardiovascular effects, craniofacial dysmorphism, microphthalmia, cleft lip and palate, mental retardation.	Isotretinoin exposure before pregnancy is not a risk because the drug is not stored in tissue. Etretinate has a long half-life and effects occur long after drug is discontinued. Topical application does not have a known risk.

TERATOLOGY

Agent	Effects	Comments
Cytomegalovirus	Hydrocephaly, microcephaly, chorioretinitis, cerebral calcifications, symmetric intrauterine growth restriction, microcephalus, brain damage, mental retardation, hearing loss.	Most common congenital infection. Congenital infection rate is 40% after primary infection and 14% after recurrent infection. Of infected infants, physical effects as listed are present in 20% after primary infection and 8% after secondary infection. No effective therapy exists.
Rubella	Microcephaly, mental retardation, cataracts, deafness, congenital heart disease; all organs may be affected.	Malformation rate is 50% if the mother is infected during first trimester. Rate of severe permanent organ damage decreases to 6% by midpregnancy. Immunization of children and nonpregnant adults is necessary for prevention. Immunization is not recommended during pregnancy, but the live attenuated vaccine virus has not been shown to cause the malformations of congenital rubella syndrome.
Syphilis	If severe infection, fetal demise with hydrops; if mild, detectable abnormalities of skin, teeth, and bones.	Penicillin treatment is effective for *Treponema pallidum* eradication to prevent progression of damage. Severity of fetal damage depends on duration of fetal infection; damage is worse if infection is greater than 20 weeks. Prevalence is increasing; need to rule out other sexually transmitted diseases.
Toxoplasmosis	Possible effects on all systems but particularly central nervous system, microcephaly, hydrocephaly, cerebral calcifications. Chorioretinitis is most common. Severity of manifestations depends on duration of disease.	Low prevalence during pregnancy (0.1-0.5%); initial maternal infection must occur during pregnancy to place fetus at risk. *Toxoplasma gondii* is transmitted to humans by raw meat or exposure to infected cat feces. In the first trimester, the incidence of fetal infection is as low as 9% and increases to approximately 59% in the third trimester. The severity of congenital infection is greater in the first trimester than at the end of gestation. Treat with pyrimethamine, sulfadiazine, or spiramycin.
Varicella	Possible effects on all organs, including skin scarring, chorioretinitis, cataracts, microcephaly, hypoplasia of the hands and feet, and muscle atrophy.	Risk of congenital varicella is low, approximately 2-3% and occurs between 7 and 21 weeks of gestation. Varicella-zoster immune globulin is available regionally for newborns exposed in utero during last 4-7 days of gestation. No effect from herpes zoster.
Radiation	Microcephaly, mental retardation.	Medical diagnostic radiation delivering less than 0.05 Gy to the fetus has no teratogenic risk. Estimated fetal exposure of common radiologic procedures is 0.01 Gy or less (e.g., intravenous pyelography, 0.0041 Gy). NOTE: 1 Gray (Gy) = 100 rad. See also page 81.

Source: American College of Obstetricians and Gynecologists. *Teratology*. ACOG Educational Bulletin, Number 236, April 1997. Copyright 1997 American College of Obstetricians and Gynecologists. Reproduced with permission.

ULTRASOUND PRINCIPLES

Indications for Ultrasonography During Pregnancy

- estimation of gestational age
- evaluation of fetal growth
- vaginal bleeding of undetermined etiology in pregnancy
- determination of fetal presentation
- suspected multiple gestation
- amniocentesis
- size/date discrepancy
- pelvic mass
- suspected molar gestation
- adjunct to cervical cerclage placement
- suspected ectopic pregnancy
- suspected fetal death
- suspected uterine abnormality
- IUD localization
- biophysical profile
- suspected abruption
- external cephalic version
- suspected polyhydramnios or oligohydramnios
- estimation of fetal weight/presentation in preterm labor or PROM
- abnormal MSAFP
- follow-up on fetal anomaly
- follow-up on placental location in previously identified previa
- history of previous congenital anomaly
- serial evaluation of growth in multiple gestation
- evaluation of fetal condition in late registrants for prenatal care

Adapted from U.S. Department of Health and Human Services. Diagnostic ultrasound in pregnancy. National Institutes of Health publication no. 84-667. Bethesda, Maryland: National Institutes of Health, 1984.

First Trimester Ultrasonography

- gestational sac location
- identification of embryo
- crown-rump length
- fetal number
- presence of cardiac activity
- evaluation of the uterus, adnexa and cervix

Second Trimester Ultrasonography

- fetal number
- fetal presentation
- placental localization
- amniotic fluid volume
- detection and evaluation of maternal pelvic masses
- gestational dating using at least two fetal parameters
- documentation of fetal cardiac activity (including rate and rhythm)
- anatomic survey
    - head: plane of BPD/HC, midline of brain, posterior fossa
    - spine: sagittal and coronal views
    - heart: 4 chamber view
    - abdomen: fetal bladder, kidneys, stomach, and umbilical cord insertion

ULTRASOUND

FIRST TRIMESTER ULTRASOUND APPEARANCE
Early Landmarks by Endovaginal Sonography

4 weeks	Choriodecidual thickening; chorionic sac
5 weeks	Chorionic sac (5-15 mm); yolk sac
6 weeks	Yolk sac/embryo; detectable heart motion
7 weeks	Embryo/fetal movement; prominent rhombencephalon
8 weeks	Physiologic bowel herniation; arms, legs

Source: Fleischer AC, Rao BK and Kepple DM. Normal Early Pregnancy. In Fleischer AC and Kepple DM editors. *Transvaginal Sonography: A Clinical Atlas.* Philadelphia: J.B. Lippincott, 1992. Reproduced with permission.

Landmarks and β-hCG Levels
• gestational sac should be visualized by 1000-1200 mIU/mL
• yolk sac should be visualized by 7,200 mIU/mL
• embryo with cardiac activity should be visualized by 10,800 mIU/mL

Embryo
• cardiac activity may be visible as soon as fetal pole identified
• if embryo is 3-5 mm but no cardiac activity, repeat sonogram in 3-5 days to evaluate viability
• fetal heart rate starts at 80-100 bpm then increases at 7-9 weeks
• embryo grows 1 mm/day

Outcome
• fetal loss rate after finding cardiac activity is 5%
• loss rate is significantly higher in patients reporting recurrent spontaneous abortion

Exceptions to Performing a Complete Ultrasound Survey
• placental localization in cases of antepartum hemorrhage or prior to cesarean
• determination of fetal lie or presentation in labor
• estimation of fetal size or weight in emergency situation
• determination of multiple gestation
• ultrasound guided amniocentesis
• external cephalic version
• confirmation of cardiac activity
• biophysical profile in patient who has had a prior basic or targeted ultrasound
• amniotic fluid volume
• previous second trimester basic and/or targeted ultrasound

FETAL ANATOMIC LANDMARKS

Legend

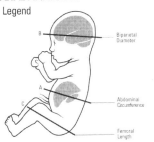

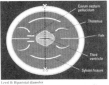

Level B: Biparietal diameter

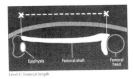

Level C: Femoral length

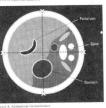

Level A: Abdominal circumference

INTRACRANIAL ANATOMY

Legend

Level A: Lateral Ventricles

Level B: Biparietal diameter

Level C: Cerebellum

Level D: Posterior fossa

ULTRASOUND

ENDOVAGINAL ULTRASONOGRAPHY

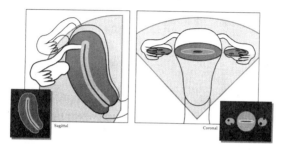

Sagittal   Coronal

Reproduced with permission from Advanced Technology Laboratories (ATL), Bothell, Washington.
Clinical source: Kris M. Holoska, RDMS, Antenatal Testing Unit, Pennsylvania Hospital, Philadelphia, Pennsylvania.

ANATOMY

Uterus
• check the cervix with the probe pulled back slightly
• scan and measure the size of the uterus in the sagittal and coronal views
• check for posterior masses and fluid in the cul-de-sac

Ovaries
• usually adjacent to the femoral vessels
• check for free fluid around the tubes and ovaries
• scan completely through the ovary in two planes
• normal ovarian volume is 6-14 cm^3

Endometrium
• begins to thicken during the follicular phase of the cycle
• around ovulation can usually identify a "triple line"
• during the secretory phase of the cycle the endometrium is thick (8-12 mm) and echogenic
• should not measure > 6-8 mm in postmenopausal patients
• abnormalities may indicate hyperplasia or neoplasia

FETAL ECHOCARDIOGRAPHY

Standard Fetal Echocardiographic Views and What to See

1. General
First determine situs:
- Identify fetal position
- Locate fetal stomach and other abdominal organs
- Verify relationship of fetal stomach to fetal heart
- Apex of heart should be to the left

2. Four-Chamber
Obtain a four-chamber view. Locate and verify:
- An intact interventricular septum
- Right and left atria approximately the same size
- Right and left ventricles approximately equal sizes
- Free movement of mitral and tricuspid valves
- Foramen ovale flap in left atrium

3. Long Axis Left Ventricle
Obtain the long axis view of the left ventricle.
Locate and verify:
- Intact interventricular septum
- Continuity of the ascending aorta with:
  -Mitral valve posterior
  -Interventricular septum anterior

4. Short Axis of Great Vessels
Obtain the short axis view of the great vessels. Locate:
- Pulmonary artery which should exit the anterior (right) ventricle and bifurcate

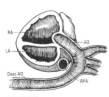

5. Aortic Arch
Locate the aortic arch and verify that:
- The aorta exits from the posterior (left) ventricle (not shown)
- Three head and neck vessels should branch from the aorta

6. Pulmonary Artery-Ductus Arteriosus
Locate the descending aorta and confirm:
- Continuity of the ductus arteriosus with the descending aorta

CLINICAL SOURCE:
Joshua A. Copel M.D., Director, Division of Maternal-Fetal Medicine, Department of Obstetrics and Gynecology, Yale University School of Medicine, New Haven, CT

ULTRASOUND

ULTRASOUND MEASUREMENTS

Weeks	BPD (mm)	HC (mm)	FL (mm)	AC (mm)	Weeks	BPD (mm)	HC (mm)	FL (mm)	AC (mm)
12	15	56	7	51	29	72	266	55	248
13	19	72	10	63	30	75	275	57	258
14	24	89	14	75	31	77	283	60	269
15	28	105	17	87	32	80	290	62	279
16	32	120	20	100	33	82	298	64	290
17	36	135	23	112	34	85	305	66	300
18	39	149	26	124	35	87	312	68	311
19	43	162	29	135	36	89	319	70	321
20	46	175	32	147	37	91	326	72	331
21	50	187	35	159	38	93	333	74	341
22	53	198	37	170	39	96	339	76	351
23	56	209	40	182	40	98	345	78	361
24	59	220	43	193	41	100	351	80	371
25	62	230	45	204					
26	64	239	48	215					
27	67	249	50	226					
28	70	258	53	237					

$$\text{Cranial Index} = \frac{\text{BPD (outer-outer)}}{\text{AP}}$$

CI < 74 = Dolichocephalic

$$HC = (BPD + OFC + 0.2)\,1.57$$

Abdominal Circumference

Biparietal Diameter (cm)	17	18	19	20	21	22	23	24	25	26	27
5.0	434	468	505	545	587	633	683	737	794	857	924
5.2	459	495	533	574	618	666	717	772	832	896	965
5.4	486	522	562	605	650	700	753	810	871	937	1008
5.6	513	552	593	637	684	735	790	849	912	980	1053
5.8	543	583	625	671	720	773	829	890	955	1025	1100
6.0	574	615	659	707	758	812	870	933	1000	1072	1149
6.2	607	650	696	745	797	853	913	978	1047	1121	1200
6.4	642	686	734	784	839	897	959	1025	1096	1172	1253
6.6	678	725	774	826	882	942	1006	1075	1148	1226	1309
6.8	717	765	816	870	928	990	1056	1127	1202	1282	1367
7.0	758	808	861	917	977	1041	1109	1181	1258	1340	1428
7.2	802	853	908	966	1028	1094	1164	1238	1317	1402	1491
7.4	848	901	958	1018	1081	1149	1221	1298	1379	1466	1558
7.6	896	952	1010	1072	1138	1208	1282	1361	1444	1533	1627
7.8	948	1005	1065	1129	1197	1269	1346	1426	1512	1603	1700
8.0	1002	1061	1124	1190	1260	1334	1412	1495	1583	1677	1775
8.2	1060	1121	1185	1253	1325	1402	1482	1568	1658	1753	1854
8.4	1120	1183	1250	1320	1395	1473	1556	1643	1736	1834	1937
8.6	1185	1250	1318	1391	1467	1548	1633	1723	1818	1918	2023
8.8	1252	1320	1391	1465	1544	1627	1714	1806	1903	2005	2113
9.0	1324	1394	1467	1544	1624	1710	1799	1893	1993	2097	2207
9.2	1400	1472	1547	1626	1709	1797	1888	1985	2087	2193	2305
9.4	1480	1554	1632	1713	1798	1888	1962	2081	2185	2294	2408
9.6	1565	1641	1721	1805	1892	1984	2080	2182	2287	2399	2515
9.8	1655	1733	1815	1901	1991	2085	2184	2287	2395	2508	2627
10.0	1750	1830	1915	2003	2095	2191	2292	2398	2508	2623	2744

Sources: Hadlock FP, Deter RL, Harrist RB, et al. Estimating fetal age: computer-assisted analysis of multiple fetal growth parameters. Radiology. 1984;152(2):497-501. Robinson HP, Fleming JE. A critical evaluation of sonar "crown-rump length" measurements. Br J Obstet Gynaecol. 1975;82(9):702-10. Shepard MJ, Richards VA, Berkowitz RL, et al. An evaluation of two equations for predicting fetal weight by ultrasound. Am J Obstet Gynecol. 1982;142(1):47-54. Williams RL, Creasy RK, Cunningham GC, et al. Fetal growth and perinatal viability in California. Obstet Gynecol. 1982;59(5):624-32.

ULTRASOUND MEASUREMENTS

Crown - Rump Length

CRL (mm)	Weeks	CRL (mm)	Weeks
8	6.8	42	11.1
10	7.2	44	11.3
12	7.6	46	11.5
14	7.9	48	11.7
16	8.2	50	11.9
18	8.5	52	12.0
20	8.8	54	12.2
22	9.0	56	12.4
24	9.3	58	12.5
26	9.5	60	12.7
28	9.7	62	12.8
30	9.9	64	13.0
32	10.2	66	13.1
34	10.4	68	13.3
36	10.6	70	13.4
38	10.8	72	13.5
40	11.0	74	13.7
		76	13.8

Fetal Weight (grams)

	50th %	10th %	90th %
21	513	320	746
22	513	320	746
23	589	365	861
24	675	417	989
25	773	477	1132
26	882	546	1289
27	1005	627	1463
28	1143	720	1653
29	1298	829	1809
30	1484	955	2136
31	1695	1100	2402
32	1920	1284	2673
33	2155	1499	2910
34	2394	1728	3132
35	2628	1974	3333
36	2849	2224	3521
37	3052	2455	3706
38	3227	2642	3867
39	3364	2790	3994
40	3462	2891	4080
41	3589	3011	4185

Abdominal Circumference (cm)

Biparietal Diameter

28	29	30	31	32	33	34	35	36	37	38	39	40
996	1074	1159	1249	1347	1453	1567	1689	1822	1965	2119	2285	2464
1039	1119	1206	1299	1389	1506	1623	1748	1882	2027	2183	2352	2533
1084	1166	1255	1350	1452	1562	1680	1808	1945	2092	2250	2421	2604
1131	1215	1306	1403	1507	1620	1740	1870	2009	2158	2319	2492	2677
1180	1266	1359	1458	1565	1679	1802	1934	2075	2227	2390	2565	2753
1231	1319	1414	1516	1625	1741	1866	2001	2144	2298	2463	2640	2830
1284	1375	1472	1576	1687	1806	1933	2069	2215	2371	2539	2718	2909
1340	1433	1532	1638	1751	1872	2002	2140	2289	2447	2616	2797	2991
1398	1493	1594	1702	1818	1941	2073	2214	2364	2525	2696	2880	3075
1458	1555	1659	1769	1887	2013	2147	2290	2443	2605	2779	2964	3161
1521	1621	1726	1839	1959	2087	2224	2369	2524	2688	2864	3051	3250
1587	1689	1797	1912	2034	2164	2303	2450	2607	2774	2952	3141	3342
1656	1759	1870	1987	2112	2244	2385	2534	2693	2862	3042	3233	3435
1727	1833	1946	2065	2192	2327	2470	2622	2783	2954	3135	3328	3532
1802	1910	2025	2147	2276	2413	2558	2712	2875	3048	3231	3425	3631
1880	1990	2107	2231	2363	2502	2649	2805	2970	3145	3330	3526	3733
1961	2074	2193	2319	2453	2594	2743	2901	3068	3245	3432	3629	3838
2046	2161	2282	2411	2547	2690	2841	3001	3170	3348	3537	3736	3946
2134	2252	2375	2506	2644	2789	2942	3104	3275	3455	3645	3845	4057
2227	2346	2472	2605	2745	2892	3047	3211	3383	3565	3756	3958	4171
2323	2445	2573	2707	2849	2999	3156	3321	3495	3679	3871	4074	4288
2423	2547	2677	2814	2958	3109	3268	3435	3611	3796	3990	4194	4408
2528	2654	2786	2925	3071	3224	3385	3554	3731	3917	4112	4317	4532
2637	2765	2900	3041	3188	3343	3505	3676	3854	4041	4238	4444	4659
2751	2881	3018	3160	3310	3466	3630	3802	3982	4170	4367	4579	4790
2870	3002	3141	3285	3436	3594	3760	3933	4114	4303	4501	4708	4925

ULTRASOUND

METRIC/ENGLISH WEIGHT CONVERSION

OUNCES →

POUNDS ↓	15	14	13	12	11	10	9	8	7	6	5	4	3	2	1	0
0	425	397	369	340	312	283	255	227	198	170	142	113	85	57	28	
1	879	850	822	794	765	737	709	680	652	624	595	567	539	510	482	454
2	1332	1304	1276	1247	1219	1191	1162	1134	1106	1077	1049	1021	992	964	936	907
3	1786	1758	1729	1701	1673	1644	1616	1588	1559	1531	1503	1474	1446	1417	1389	1361
4	2240	2211	2183	2155	2126	2098	2070	2041	2013	1984	1956	1928	1899	1871	1843	1814
5	2693	2665	2637	2608	2580	2551	2523	2495	2466	2438	2410	2381	2353	2325	2296	2268
6	3147	3118	3090	3062	3033	3005	2977	2948	2920	2892	2863	2835	2807	2778	2750	2722
7	3600	3572	3544	3515	3487	3459	3430	3402	3374	3345	3317	3289	3260	3232	3203	3175
8	4054	4026	3997	3969	3941	3912	3884	3856	3827	3799	3770	3742	3714	3685	3657	3629
9	4508	4479	4451	4423	4394	4366	4337	4309	4281	4252	4224	4196	4167	4139	4111	4082
10	4961	4933	4904	4876	4848	4819	4791	4763	4734	4706	4678	4649	4621	4593	4564	4536
11	5415	5386	5358	5330	5301	5273	5245	5216	5188	5160	5131	5103	5075	5046	5018	4990
12	5868	5840	5812	5783	5755	5727	5698	5670	5642	5613	5585	5557	5528	5500	5471	5443
13	6322	6294	6265	6237	6209	6180	6152	6123	6095	6067	6038	6010	5982	5953	5925	5897
14	6775	6747	6719	6690	6662	6634	6605	6577	6549	6520	6492	6464	6435	6407	6379	6350

POUNDS

CONTRACEPTIVE CHOICES

Method	% of Women Experiencing an Accidental Pregnancy within the First Year of Use		% of Women Continuing Use at 1 Year[3]
	Typical Use[1]	Perfect Use[2]	
No method[4]	85	85	
Spermicides[5]	26	6	40
Periodic Abstinence	25		63
Calendar		9	
Ovulation method		3	
Symptothermal[6]		2	
Post-ovulation		1	
Cervical cap[7]			
Parous women	40	26	42
Nulliparous women	20	9	56
Sponge			
Parous women	40	20	42
Nulliparous women	20	9	56
Diaphragm[7]	20	6	56
Withdrawal	19	4	
Condom[8]			
Female (Reality)	21	5	56
Male	14	3	61
Contraceptive Pill	5		71
Progestin only		0.5	
Combination		0.1	
IUD			
Progesterone IUD	2	1.5	81
Copper T 380A	0.8	0.6	78
LNG 20	0.1	0.1	81
Depo-Provera	0.3	0.3	70
Norplant & Norplant II	0.05	0.05	88
Female Sterilization	0.4	0.4	100
Male Sterilization	0.15	0.10	100

Emergency contraceptive pills: Treatment initiated within 72 hours after unprotected intercourse reduces the risk of pregnancy by at least 75%.[9]

Lactational amenorrhea method: LAM is a highly effective, temporary method of contraception.[10]

[1] Among typical couples who initiate use of a method (not necessarily for the first time), the percentage who experience an accidental pregnancy during the first year if they do not stop use for any other reason.
[2] Among couples who initiate use of a method (not necessarily for the first time) and who use it perfectly (both consistently and correctly), the percentage who experience an accidental pregnancy during the first year if they do not stop use for any other reason.
[3] Among couples attempting to avoid pregnancy, the percentage who continue to use a method for 1 year.
[4] The percentages becoming pregnant in the typical use and perfect use columns are based on data from populations where contraception is not used and from women who cease using contraception in order to become pregnant. Among such populations, about 89% become pregnant within 1 year. This estimate was lowered slightly (to 85%) to represent the percentage who would become pregnant within 1 year among women now relying on reversible methods of contraception if they abandoned contraception altogether.
[5] Foams, creams, gels, vaginal suppositories, and vaginal film.
[6] Cervical mucus (ovulation) method supplemented by calendar in the pre-ovulatory and basal body temperature in the post-ovulatory phases.
[7] With spermicidal cream or jelly.
[8] Without spermicides.
[9] The treatment schedule is one dose within 72 hours after unprotected intercourse, and a second dose 12 hours after the first dose.
[10] However, to maintain effective protection against pregnancy, another method of contraception must be used as soon as menstruation resumes, the frequency or duration of breastfeeds is reduced, bottle feeds are introduced, or the baby reaches 6 months of age.

Source: Trussell J. Contraceptive efficacy. In Hatcher RA, Trussell J, Stewart FH et al. *Contraceptive Technology: Seventeenth Revised Edition.* New York, NY: Irvington Publishers, 1998.

GYNECOLOGY

BARRIER CONTRACEPTIVES
Diaphragm
• safe method with rare side effects
• UTI twice as common
• reduces rate of STD's
• successful fitting is crucial to efficacy
• insert no longer than 6 hr prior to coitus
• remove 6-24 hr after coitus
• use with spermicide
• assess fit annually

Cervical Cap (Prentif)
• safe method with rare side effects
• only 4 sizes and harder to place
• insert 20 min to 4 hours prior to coitus
• successful fitting is crucial to efficacy
• can leave in place for 24-36 hours

Spermicides
• Nonoxynol-9, Octoxynol-9, Mefegol
• proven STD protection
• apply 10-30 min prior to coitus
• high failure rate

Condoms
• 6 billion used worldwide annually
• latex condoms 0.3-0.8 mm thick
• natural skin condoms do **not** protect against HIV
  and other STD's
• do not use with oil-based lubricants
• inconsistent use accounts for most failures

ORAL CONTRACEPTIVES

Contraindications

Absolute
- pregnancy
- previous or active thromboembolic disease
- undiagnosed genital bleeding
- smoking and age 35
- estrogen dependent neoplasm
- hepatoma

Relative
- hypertension
- diabetes
- gallbladder disease
- obesity
- migraines

Advantages
- excellent form of contraception
- decreased incidence in ovarian and endometrial carcinoma
- decreased monthly menstrual flow
- decreased dysmenorrhea
- decreased incidence of PID
- decreased incidence of benign breast disease

Disadvantages
- breakthrough bleeding
- weight gain
- depression
- nausea
- hypertension (rare)

Management
- start on 1st Sunday of cycle (monophasics) or 1st day of period (triphasics)
- protected from pregnancy after 5 days
- if miss 1 pill → take missed pill as soon as possible, take next pill at usual time
- if miss 2 pills during 1st two weeks → take 2 pills as soon as possible, then 2 pills the next
     day, then return to usual schedule but use additional barrier contraception for that month
- if miss 2 pills during 3rd week or 3 pills at any time during month then immediately start a new
     pack without having a pill-free interval and use back-up method for 7 days
- breakthrough bleeding (BTB) common in 1st 3 months
    - if BTB still a problem after that then change to different OC

GYNECOLOGY

COMMON ORAL CONTRACEPTIVES

Drug	Manufacturer	Estrogen (mcg)	Progestin (mg)
Ovral Ogestrel-28	Wyeth-Ayerst Watson	ethinyl estradiol (50)	norgestrel (0.5)
Ovcon 50	Warner Chilcott	ethinyl estradiol (50)	norethindrone (1)
Zovia 1/50E	Watson	ethinyl estradiol (50)	ethynodiol diacetate (1)
Genora 1/50 Necon 1/50 Nelova 1/50 Norinyl 1/50	Physicians Total Care Watson Warner Chilcott Watson	mestranol (50)	norethindrone (1)
Ovcon 35	Warner Chilcott	ethinyl estradiol (35)	norethindrone (0.4)
Modicon Brevicon Necon 0.5/35E	Ortho-McNeil Watson Watson	ethinyl estradiol (35)	norethindrone (0.5)
Nelova 10/11	Warner Chilcott	ethinyl estradiol (35)	norethindrone (0.5,1)
Ortho-Novum 1/35 Genora 1/35 Necon 1/35 Nelova 1/35 Norinyl 1/35	Ortho-McNeil Physicians Total Care Watson Warner Chilcott Watson	ethinyl estradiol (35)	norethindrone (1)
Ortho-Cyclen	Ortho-McNeil	ethinyl estradiol (35)	norgestimate (0.25)
Demulen 1/35 Zovia 1/35E	Searle Watson	ethinyl estradiol (35)	ethynodiol diacetate (1)
Loestrin 1.5/30	Parke-Davis	ethinyl estradiol (30)	norethindrone acetate (1.5)
Levlen 21 Levora Nordette	Berlex Watson Wyeth-Ayerst	ethinyl estradiol (30)	levonorgestrel (0.15)
Lo/Ovral Low-Ogestrel	Wyeth-Ayerst Watson	ethinyl estradiol (30)	norgestrel (0.3)
Ortho-Cept Desogen 28	Ortho-McNeil Organon	ethinyl estradiol (30)	desogestrel (0.15)
Alesse Levlite	Wyeth-Ayerst Berlex	ethinyl estradiol (20)	levonorgestrel (0.1)
Loestrin 1/20	Parke-Davis	ethinyl estradiol (20)	norethindrone acetate (1)

COMMON ORAL CONTRACEPTIVES (CONT.)

Drug	Manufacturer	Estrogen (mcg)	Progestin (mg)
Multiphasic Combinations			
Tri-Levlen Tri-Phasil Trivora-28	Berlex Wyeth-Ayerst Watson	ethinyl estradiol (30, 40, 30)	levonorgestrel (0.05, 0.075, 0.125)
Estrostep 28	Parke-Davis	ethinyl estradiol (20, 30, 35)	norethindrone acetate (1)
Ortho Tri-Cyclen	Ortho-McNeil	ethinyl estradiol (35)	norgestimate (0.18, 0.215, 0.25)
Tri-Norinyl	Watson	ethinyl estradiol (35)	norethindrone (0.5, 1, 0.5)
Ortho-Novum 7/7/7	Ortho-McNeil	ethinyl estradiol (35)	norethindrone (0.5, 0.75, 1)
Ortho-Novum 10/11 Jenest-28 Necon 10/11	Ortho-McNeil Organon Watson	ethinyl estradiol (35)	norethindrone (0.5, 1)
Mircette	Organon	ethinyl estradiol (20, 0, 10)	desogestrel (0.15)
Cyclessa	Organon	ethinyl estradiol (25)	desogestrel (0.1, 0.125, 0.15)
Progestin Only			
Ovrette	Wyeth-Ayerst	none	norgestrel (0.075)
Micronor Nor-QD	Ortho-McNeil Watson	none	norethindrone (0.35)

GYNECOLOGY

ORAL CONTRACEPTIVE GUIDELINES

Practice Guidelines for OC Selection: Summary

1=First Choice; combination formulations containing 30-35 mcg of ethinyl estradiol (EE) except where noted. See footnotes.
2=Second Choice; combination formulations containing 30-35 mcg of ethinyl estradiol (EE) except where noted. See footnotes.

Patient Characteristics	Progestin Androgenic Activity		
	Low	Medium	High

	Norgestimate
	Desogestrel
	Norethindrone 0.4-0.5 mg
	  monophasic
		Levonorgestrel triphasic
		Norethindrone 1 mg
		  monophasic or triphasic
		Norethindrone acetate 1 mg
		Ethynodiol diacetate 1 mg
			Norgestrel 0.3 mg
			Norethindrone acetate 1.5-2.5 mg
			Levonorgestrel 0.15 mg

General Formulation Selections for Women Initiating OC Use			
New start (all women except where noted in Tables 4 and 5)	1	2	
Adolescent	1	2	
Perimenopause	1	2	
Postpartum (lactating)	If no supplemental feedings and no menses, conception unlikely for 2-3 months; if OC desired, progestin-only pill recommended 6 weeks after delivery. Replace with combination pill when supplemental feeding introduced.		
Postpartum (non-lactating) (start at 2 weeks)	1	2	
Formulation Selections in Minimizing or Managing Unwanted OC Side Effects			
BTB	1[a]	1[a]	
Weight gain	1	2	
Acne/hirsutism	1	2	
Headaches/common migraine	1[b,c]	2	
Nausea	1[b,d]	2	
Breast tenderness	1[b,d]	2	
Mood change	1[b]	2	
Formulation Selections in Minimizing or Managing OC Adverse Effects			
Adverse lipid/lipoprotein effects (except hypertriglyceridemia, see table 4)	1	2	
Adverse carbohydrate effects	No current formulations have a clinically significant effect on glucose metabolism		
Adverse thrombotic effects	Thrombotic effects are primarily related to the dose of the estrogen component; use OC containing less than 50 mcg estrogen or other method		

[a]The lowest incidence of BTB appears to be with formulations containing either levonorgestrel, norgestimate, or desogestrel. If BTB persists after switching from one such formulation to another - and if poor compliance, infection, and other potential problems have been ruled out - placement of the patient on a preparation containing 50 mcg estrogen may be considered.

[a]A formulation containing a progestin with low androgenic activity remains the agent of choice, but evidence for a clear advantage in this parameter is lacking; if the problem persists, switching to a pill containing a different type of progestin may be beneficial in some individuals.

[c]If headache occurs exclusively during the pill-free interval, use daily, continuous, combined OCs to avoid cyclicity.

[d]This effect is largely estrogenic and infrequent with low estrogen dose OCs. If the problem persists, a 20 mcg EE formulation may be tried.

ORAL CONTRACEPTIVE GUIDELINES (CONT.)

Practice Guidelines for OC Selection: Summary

1=First Choice; combination formulations containing 30-35 mcg of ethinyl estradiol (EE) except where noted. See footnotes.
2=Second Choice; combination formulations containing 30-35 mcg of ethinyl estradiol (EE) except where noted. See footnotes.

Patient Characteristics	Progestin Androgenic Activity		
	Low	Medium	High
	Norgestimate Desogestrel Norethindrone 0.4-0.5 mg	Levonorgesrel triphasic Norethindrone 1 mg (monophasic or triphasic) Norethindrone acetate 1 mg Ethynodiol diacetate 1 mg	Norgestrel 0.3 mg Norethindrone acetate 1.5-2.5 mg Levonorgesrel 0.15 mg
Formulation Selections for Women with Medical Conditions			
Acne/hirsutism	1	2	
Obesity	1	2	
History of vascular disease (eg, thromboembolism, CAD)	Contraindication		
Hypertension (uncontrolled)	Contraindication		
Hypertension (controlled or history of pregnancy-induced)	1	2	
Hypercholesterolemia	1	2	
Hypertriglyceridemia	OCs contraindicated above 350-600 mg/dL, depending on panel member's view and presence/absence of other factors (eg, low HDL); with mild elevations, a norgestimate-containing OC may be preferred		
Smoker older than 35 years of age	Contraindication		
Smoker 30-35 years of age	1[a]	1 (less than 50 mcg estrogen)	
Heavy smoker less than 30 years of age	1[a]	1 (less than 50 mcg estrogen)	
Family history of CHD	1	2	
Classic migraine	Contraindication		
Common migraine	1[b]	2	
Depression	1[b]	2	
Family history of breast cancer	1[b,c]	2	
Personal history of breast cancer	Contraindication		
Benign breast disease	1[b,d]	2	
Diabetes/gestational diabetes	1[b]	2	
Antiepileptic drug use	Formulation containing 50 mcg estrogen may be preferable		
Family history of ovarian cancer	1	2	
Sickle cell	1	2	
Prosthetic heart valve	1	2	
Anticoagulant use	1	2	
Mitral valve prolapse	1	2	

[a]There is no epidemiologic evidence indicating that there is a difference in risk of venous thrombosis with 20 mcg EE and 30-35 mcg EE OCs in smokers as well as nonsmokers.
[a]A formulation containing a progestin with low androgenic activity remains the agent of choice, but evidence for a clear advantage in this parameter is lacking; if the problem persists, switching to a pill containing a different type of progestin may be beneficial in some individuals.
[c]A formulation containing a progestin with low androgenic activity remains the agent of choice, but there is no evidence that any particular OC formulation is preferable in women with a family history of breast cancer.
[d] OCs generally protect against the development of benign breast disease; a formulation containing a progestin with low androgenic activity remains the agent of first choice.

GYNECOLOGY

ORAL CONTRACEPTIVE GUIDELINES (CONT.)

Practice Guidelines for OC Selection: Summary

1=First Choice; combination formulations containing 30-35 mcg of ethinyl estradiol (EE) except where noted. See footnotes.
2=Second Choice; combination formulations containing 30-35 mcg of ethinyl estradiol (EE) except where noted. See footnotes.
In some instances there are two first choices.

Patient Characteristics	Progestin Androgenic Activity		
	Low	**Medium**	**High**
	Norgestimate Desogestrel Norethindrone 0.4-0.5 mg monophasic	Levonorgestrel triphasic Norethindrone 1 mg (monophasic or triphasic) Norethindrone acetate 1 mg Ethynodiol diacetate 1 mg	Norgestrel 0.3 mg Norethindrone acetate 1.5-2.5 mg Levonorgestrel 0.15 mg
Formulation Selections in Women for Whom OCs Are Being Considered in Some Measure for Therapeutic Purposes			
Ovulatory dysfunctional uterine bleeding	1	2	
Persistent anovulation	1	2	
Premature ovarian failure	1	2	
Dysmenorrhea	1[a,b]	1[a,b]	
Functional ovarian cysts	1 (monophasic only)		2 (monophasic only)
Mittelschmerz	1[a]	2	
Endometriosis (pain)		1 (monophasic continuous)	2 (monophasic continuous)
Bleeding with blood dyscrasias		1 (continuous)	2 (continuous)

[a]A formulation containing a progestin with low androgenic activity remains the agent of choice, but evidence for a clear advantage in this parameter is lacking; if the problem persists, switching to a pill containing a different type of progestin may be beneficial in some individuals.

[b]A formulation containing a progestin with low androgenic activity remains the agent of first choice, and may be used in combination with a prostaglandin synthetase inhibitor. If dysmenorrea persists, options include the use of an agent with higher androgenic activity plus a prostaglandin synthetae inhibitor or diagnostic tests to rule out endometriosis.

Source: Mishell DR, Darney PD, Burkman RT, Sulak PJ. Practice guidelines for OC selection:update. *Dialogues in Contraception* 1997;5(4):7-20.

EMERGENCY POST-COITAL ORAL CONTRACEPTION

Fast Facts
- safety confirmed in several large multicenter trials
- appropriate candidate is reproductive-age women within 72 hours of unprotected coitus
    - often associated with failure of barrier contraception
- treatment reduces pregnancy rate by 75% (range 55%-94%) based on published studies
    - effective pregnancy rate ~ 2%
- other option: midcycle IUD placement
    - failure rate 0.1%
- 98% of patients will menstruate by 21 days after treatment (mean 7-9 days)

Yuzpe Method and Equivalent Doses
- two doses taken 12 hours apart, with an antiemetic agent such as Tigan, Phenergan, Benadryl etc.

Drug	Manufacturer	Estrogen (mcg)	Progestin (mg)	Pills per Dose
Dedicated Products				
Preven	Gynetics	ethinyl estradiol (50)	levonorgestrel (0.25)	2 blue
Plan B	Womens Capital	none	levonorgestrel (0.75)	1 white
Combination OCs				
Ovral	Wyeth-Ayerst	ethinyl estradiol (50)	norgestrel (0.5)	2 white
Levlen 21	Berlex	ethinyl estradiol (30)	levonorgestrel (0.15)	4 light-orange
Nordette	Wyeth-Ayerst			4 light-orange
Levora	Watson			4 white
Lo/Ovral	Wyeth-Ayerst	ethinyl estradiol (30)	norgestrel (0.3)	4 white
Low-Ogestrel	Watson			4 white
Alesse	Wyeth-Ayerst	ethinyl estradiol (20)	levonorgestrel (0.1)	5 pink
Levlite	Berlex			5 pink
Tri-Levlen	Berlex	ethinyl estradiol (30)	levonorgestrel (0.125)	4 yellow
Tri-Phasil	Wyeth-Ayerst			4 yellow
Trivora-28	Watson			4 pink
Progestin Only				
Ovrette	Wyeth-Ayerst	none	norgestrel (0.075)	20 yellow pills

- check pregnancy test in 21 days if no menses

Source: Trussell J and Stewart F. An Update on Emergency Oral Contraceptives. *Dialogues in Contraception*. 1998:5(6):1-5. Reproduced with permission.

GYNECOLOGY

NORPLANT
Fast Facts
- subdermal implant system
- long acting, low dose, reversible, progestin only
- 6 capsules, 34 mm long, each with 36 mg of levonorgestrel

Mechanism of action
- suppression of LH surge at pituitary and hypothalamic level
- thickens cervical mucus
- suppresses endometrial maturation

Contraindications
Absolute
1. Active thrombophlebitis or thromboembolic disease
2. Undiagnosed genital bleeding
3. Acute liver disease
4. Benign or malignant liver tumors
5. Known or suspected breast cancer

Relative
1. Heavy cigarette smoking in patient > 35 years old
2. History of ectopic pregnancy
3. Diabetes mellitus (most studies show no effect)
4. Hypercholesterolemia
5. Severe acne
6. Hypertension
7. History of cardiovascular disease
8. Gallbladder disease
9. Severe vascular or migraine headaches
10. Severe depression
11. Chronic disease, immunocompromised patients
12. Concomitant use of medications that increase microsomal liver enzymes

Advantages
- highly effective

Year 1	0.2% (woman-years)
Year 2	0.2
Year 3	0.9
Year 4	0.5
Year 5	1.1

- rapidly reversible
- little effort needed for compliance
- can be used in patients unable to take estrogen

Disadvantages
- irregular bleeding in up to 80% of patients
- does not reduce STD risk
- requires surgical insertion and removal
- removal may require use of several different techniques

Treatment of Bleeding Abnormalities

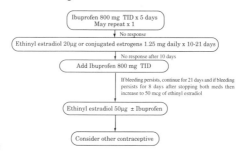

Ibuprofen 800 mg TID x 5 days
May repeat x 1

No response

Ethinyl estradiol 20µg or conjugated estrogens 1.25 mg daily x 10-21 days

No response after 10 days

Add Ibuprofen 800 mg TID

If bleeding persists, continue for 21 days and if bleeding persists for 8 days after stopping both meds then increase to 50 mcg of ethinyl estradiol

Ethinyl estradiol 50µg ± Ibuprofen

Consider other contraceptive

DEPO-PROVERA
Fast Facts
• reversible and highly effective progestin only injectable contraceptive (36)
• 150 mg IM every 3 months
• contraceptive levels maintained for 14 weeks allowing 2 week grace period
• for maximum effectiveness begin within 5 days of menses

Mechanism of Action
• blocks LH surge (significantly more than Norplant)
• thickens cervical mucus
• alters endometrium

Advantages
• highly effective (<1% failure rate)
• fewer bleeding abnormalities, higher rate of amenorrhea than Norplant
• minimizes user compliance as a source of contraceptive failure

Disadvantages
• delay in return of fertility
    • ovulation delayed for 5 months, but 70% of couples conceive within 1 year of stopping drug
    • no permanent effect on fertility
• weight gain (5 lb/year)
• slight reversible bone loss
• bleeding abnormalities
    • 2/3 of women experience irregular and possibly heavy bleeding during first 3 months
• other less common side effects (headaches, abdominal/breast bloating, mood changes)

Bleeding Patterns

	Amenorrhea (%)	1-7 days of spotting/month (%)	8-30 days of spotting/month (%)
3 months	30	25	45
6 months	40	25	35
12 months	50	25	25
24 months	65	20	15

Treatment of Bleeding Abnormalities

Ibuprofen 800 mg TID x 5 days
    ↓ Bleeding persists
Ethinyl estradiol 20µg or conjugated estrogens 1.25 mg daily x 10-21 days
    ↓ Bleeding persists
Consider other contraceptive

GYNECOLOGY

LUNELLE
Fast Facts
• reversible and highly effective estrogen and progestin injectable contraception
• 5 mg estradiol cypionate + 25 mg MPA IM every month
• ovulation resumes within 2-3 months after stopping the medication
• fewer bleeding abnormalities and shorter return of fertility than Depo-Provera
• administer within the first 5 days of onset of menses and repeat every 23-33 d
• after elective abortion, start within 7 days
• after delivery, if not breastfeeding, start within 21-28 days

Mechanism of Action
• inhibition of ovulation, but endometrium is stabilized by the estrogen resulting in minimal BTB

Advantages
• failure rate is 0.1 per 100 women-years

Disadvantages
• have heavy and early bleeding (~10-20 d after injection)
    • often improves with time
• 6% of patients will discontinue medication due to heavy bleeding
• mild weight gain 2 lb/yr

	Monthly Injectable	Oral Contraceptives	Levonorgestrel Implants	Depot MPA	IUDs
Efficacy	High	High (user-dependent)	High	High	High
Provider required to initiate	Yes	Prescription	Yes	Yes	Yes
Provider required to discontinue	No	No	Yes	No	No
Duration of protection	1 month	1 day	5 years	3 months	1-10 years
Compliance	Monthly	Daily	Every 5 years	Every 3 months	Every 1-10 years
Privacy	Yes	Pill pack	Seen or felt by some women	Yes	String may be felt by partner
Rapid return of fertility	Yes	Yes	Yes	No	Yes
Regular cycles	Yes	Yes	Sometimes	No	Yes
Amenorrhea	Uncommon	Uncommon	Sometimes	Common	Variable (common in levonorgestrel IUD)

Source: Leonhardt KK. 2001 Guide to Contraceptive Management. *Ob/Gyn Special Edition*. 2001; 4:17-22. Adapted from Shulman LP. Monthly contraceptive injection. *The Female Patient*. 2000;25:14-20.

GYNECOLOGY

INTRAUTERINE DEVICE (IUD)

Fast Facts
• most widely used reversible contraceptive in the world
• <1% of US couples use this excellent method of contraception
• 3 IUD choices now available in the US: copper IUD, progesterone IUD, levonorgestrel IUD

Mechanism of Action
• sterile inflammatory reaction to foreign body
• marked impairment of sperm action
• the IUD is not an abortifacient

Contraindications

1. Pregnancy or suspected pregnancy
2. Abnormalities of the uterus
3. Acute PID or h/o PID
4. Postpartum endometritis or infected TAB/SAB in past 3 months
5. Known or suspected uterine or cervical malignancy
6. Untreated cervicitis or vaginitis
7. Wilson's disease (Copper IUD)
8. Copper allergy (Copper IUD)
9. History of ectopic pregnancy
10. Multiple sexual partners
11. Immunocompromised state
12. Genital actinomycosis

Five-Year Cumulative Pregnancy Rates and Side Effects Leading to Discontinuation of IUD

Side Effect	Levonorgestrel IUD	Copper IUD
Pregnancy	0.5%	5.9%
Bleeding problems	13.7%	20.9%
Amenorrhea	6.0%	0%
Hormonal side effects	12.1%	2.0%
Pelvic inflammatory disease	0.8%	2.2%

Source: Leonhardt KK. 2001 Guide to Contraceptive Management. *Ob/Gyn Special Edition.* 2001; 4:17-22. Reproduced with permission of McMahon Publishing Group.

Available IUDs

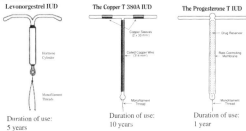

Levonorgestrel IUD
Hormone Cylinder
Monofilament Threads
Duration of use: 5 years

The Copper T 380A IUD
Copper Sleeves (2 x 33 mm²)
Coiled Copper Wire (314 mm²)
Monofilament Thread
Duration of use: 10 years

The Progesterone T IUD
Drug Reservoir
Rate-Controlling Membrane
Monofilament Thread
Duration of use: 1 year

GYNECOLOGY

TUBAL LIGATION

Fast Facts
- most frequent indication for laparoscopy in US
- preoperative counseling is essential (including failure rate)
- reversal of sterilization dependent on procedure performed
  - clips/bands have highest reversal success rates (>70%)
  - incurs increased risk of ectopic pregnancy

Laparoscopic Tubal Ligation
- performed as an interval procedure
- must clearly identify fimbria/tube
  - Falope rings applied to the round ligament do not prevent pregnancies
- perform prior to ovulation to prevent conception around the time of surgery
- most popular techniques
  - fulguration (with or without division), thermocautery, Falope rings, clips

Postpartum Tubal Ligation
- either at time of cesarean section or after vaginal delivery
- patient selection important
  - no history of pelvic adhesions
  - no history of significant PID
  - body habitus
- if patient is ambivalent, then defer to interval procedure
- empty bladder prior to performing procedure
- informed consent should always be documented
- be sure to follow up on path report to ensure the tubes were indeed excised
- Uchida/Irving have lowest failure rates

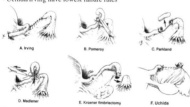

A. Irving   B. Pomeroy   C. Parkland

D. Madlener   E. Kroener fimbriectomy   F. Uchida

Source: Cunningham FG, MacDonald PC, Gant NF et al. Family planning. In: *Williams Obstetrics.* 20th ed. Stamford, Conn.: Appleton & Lange, 1997, and Depp R. Cesarean delivery and other surgical procedures. In: Gabbe SG, Niebyl JR, Simpson JL, ed. *Obstetrics: Normal and Problem Pregnancies.* 2nd ed. New York: Churchill Livingstone, 1991. Reproduced with the permission of the publishers.

Failure Rates

Method	Failures/1,000 procedures (95% CI)	
	< 30 years old	>30 years old
Bipolar coagulation	31.9 (15.2-48.7)	7.6 (1.9-13.2)
Unipolar coagulation	5.9 (0.0-17.5)	0.0
Silicone rubber-band application	11.1 (0.0-23.4)	6.9 (0.2-13.7)
Spring-clip application	7.8 (0.0-17.8)	5.8 (0.0-14.9)
Interval partial salpingectomy	14.6 (0.0-34.7)	3.7 (0.0-11.1)
Postpartum partial salpingectomy	1.2 (0.0-3.5)	1.8 (0.0-5.2)

Source: Peterson HB, Zhisen X, Hughes JM et al. The risk of ectopic pregnancy after tubal sterilization. *NEJM.* 1997; 336:762-7. Copyright 1997 Massachusetts Medical Society.

GYNECOLOGY

PAP SMEARS

Bethesda system	Classic system	Modified Papanicolaou system
Within normal limits	Normal	I
Infection (organism should be specified)	Inflammatory atypia (organism)	II
Reactive and reparative changes		IIR
Squamous cell abnormalities		
• Atypical squamous cells of undetermined significance	Squamous atypia of uncertain significance	
• Low grade squamous intraepithelial lesion (SIL)	HPV atypia Mild dysplasia CIN 1	} III
• High grade squamous intraepithelial lesion (SIL)	Moderate dysplasia CIN 2	
	Severe dysplasia } CIN 3 Carcinoma in situ	IV
• Squamous cell carcinoma	Squamous cell carcinoma	V

Suggested Evaluation

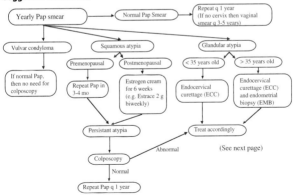

125

GYNECOLOGY

MANAGEMENT OF ABNORMAL PAP SMEARS

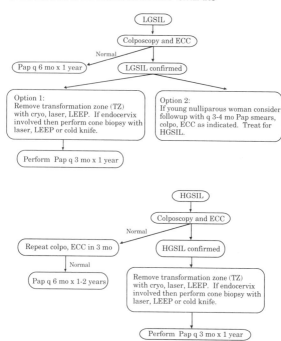

Management of dysplasia should be based on clinical evaluation.
These flow charts are only suggestions, not rigid treatment protocols.

126

LARGE LOOP EXCISION OF THE TRANSFORMATION ZONE (LLETZ)

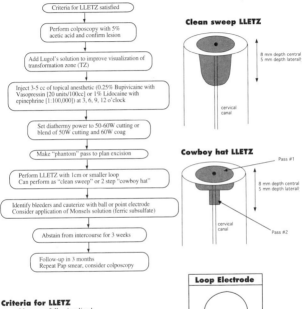

Criteria for LLETZ satisfied

Perform colposcopy with 5% acetic acid and confirm lesion

Add Lugol's solution to improve visualization of transformation zone (TZ)

Inject 3-5 cc of topical anesthetic (0.25% Bupivicaine with Vasopressin [20 units/100cc] or 1% Lidocaine with epinephrine [1:100,000]) at 3, 6, 9, 12 o'clock

Set diathermy power to 50-60W cutting or blend of 50W cutting and 60W coag

Make "phantom" pass to plan excision

Perform LLETZ with 1cm or smaller loop
Can perform as "clean sweep" or 2 step "cowboy hat"

Identify bleeders and cauterize with ball or point electrode
Consider application of Monsels solution (ferric subsulfate)

Abstain from intercourse for 3 weeks

Follow-up in 3 months
Repeat Pap smear, consider colposcopy

Clean sweep LLETZ

8 mm depth central
5 mm depth laterally

cervical canal

Cowboy hat LLETZ

Pass #1

8 mm depth central
5 mm depth laterally

cervical canal

Pass #2

Loop Electrode

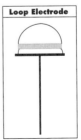

Criteria for LLETZ
• transition zone fully visualized
• no colposcopic suggestion of invasion
• colposcopic appearance correlates with Pap smear results

Results
• stenosis 3.8%
• recurrence rate 5% first year, 0.6% second year

GYNECOLOGY

DYSFUNCTIONAL UTERINE BLEEDING (DUB)

Fast Facts
- normal menses occur q 28 (mean), range 21-35 days
- normal duration 2-7 days
- normal blood loss < 80 cc
- menarche average age 13 yr
- menopause average age 51 yr
- DUB refers to any abnormal bleeding pattern for which there is no obvious cause (e.g., fibroids, polyps)

Etiology
- OCP breakthrough bleeding
- chronic anovulation
- endometrial hyperplasia
- atrophic endometrium

Evaluation
- History and physical
- β-hCG
- Consider ultrasound
- If age > 35 years, perform endometrial biopsy

Treatment
- "like treats like" i.e. if cause is hormonal then treat with hormones

Hormonal therapy
High dose estradiol (*may involve excessive risk of thromboembolic phenomenon*)

2.5 mg conjugated estrogens PO tid x 7 days then OCPs x 3 weeks **or**

OCPs qid x 7 days then daily x 3 weeks **or**

OCPs tid x 3 days, then bid x 3 days then daily

ANTICIPATE BLEEDING WHEN CHANGING DOSE

If bleeding persists:
IV conjugated estrogens (Premarin) 25 mg q 4 hr for 24 hr or until bleeding stops
      or
IM progesterone 50-100 mg

Surgical evaluation (hysteroscopy, D&C)

If bleeding persists in spite of hormonal therapy
- will provide tissue for pathologic diagnosis

NOT effective if bleeding is result of denuded endometrium

GYNECOLOGY

BACTERIAL VAGINOSIS
Fast Facts
• bacterial vaginosis is a clinical syndrome resulting from replacement of the normal vaginal flora with anaerobic bacteria in high concentrations
• associated with multiple sexual partners but unclear if this is a sexually transmitted disease
• BV is the most prevalent cause of malodorous vaginal discharge but asymptomatic in 50% of women
• several studies suggest adverse pregnancy outcomes in women with BV (preterm labor and delivery)
• presence of BV increases infectious morbidity following diagnostic (HSG) and operative procedures

Evaluation
• clinical criteria (3 of the following symptoms or signs)
  • homogeneous, white, noninflammatory discharge that coats the vaginal walls
  • the presence of clue cells on microscopic evaluation
  • a vaginal fluid pH > 4.5
  • a fishy odor of vaginal discharge before or after addition of 10% KOH (i.e. the whiff test)
• Gram stain criteria
  • alteration of the normal bacterial morphotypes
• culture is not recommended as a diagnostic tool given the non-specific nature of the results

Treatment
Nonpregnant women
Recommended regimen
Metronidazole (Flagyl), 500 mg PO bid for 7 days, or
Clindamycin cream 2%, one applicator (5 g) PV at bedtime for 10 days, or
Metronidazole vaginal gel (Metro-Gel) 0.75%, one applicator (5 g) PV bid for 5 days
Alternative regimen
Metronidazole (Flagyl), 2 g PO in a single dose, or
Clindamycin, 300 mg PO bid for 7 days

Pregnant women (2nd, 3rd trimesters)
Recommended regimen
Metronidazole (Flagyl), 250 mg PO tid for 7 days, or
Alternative regimen
Metronidazole (Flagyl), 2 g PO in a single dose, or
Clindamycin, 300 mg PO bid for 7 days, or
Metronidazole vaginal gel (Metro-Gel) 0.75%, one applicator (5 g) PV bid for 5 days (low-risk patients)

Source: 1998 Guidelines for the Treatment of Sexually Transmitted Diseases. *MMWR.* 1997; 47: RR-1.

GYNECOLOGY

TRICHOMONAS VAGINITIS

Fast Facts
- women characteristically present with a diffuse, yellow-green, malodorous discharge
- some women do not have symptoms and most men are asymptomatic
- infection with *T. vaginalis* may be associated with adverse pregnancy outcomes
  - particularly preterm PROM and preterm labor
- cure rates of 90-95% especially if treatment of male partner is included

Evaluation
- saline wet prep demonstrates motile protozoans

Treatment
Recommended regimen
Metronidazole, 2 g PO in a single dose

Alternative regimen
Metronidazole, 500 mg PO bid for 7 days, or
Metronidazole, 375 mg PO bid for 7 days

Pregnant women (2nd, 3rd trimesters)
Metronidazole, 2 g PO in a single dose

Summary

Vaginitis	pH	Hyphae	Trichomonads	Clue Cells
Bacterial vaginosis	> 4.5	absent	absent	present
Trichomoniasis	normal	absent	present	absent
Vulvovaginal candidiasis	normal	present	asent	absent

Source: 1998 Guidelines for the Treatment of Sexually Transmitted Diseases. *MMWR*. 1997; 47: RR-1.

VULVOVAGINAL CANDIDIASIS

Fast Facts

• usually caused by *C. albicans* or occasionally other *Candida* sp. or *Torulopsis* sp.
• 75% of women will experience one episode of VVC with 40-50% having two or more
• recurrent VVC is rare (<5%)
• 10-20% of women harbor yeast as normal vaginal flora

Evaluation

• clinical symptoms
    • pruritis and erythema in the vulvovaginal area
• diagnostic criteria
    • the presence of yeast or pseudohyphae on microscopic evaluation of a 10% KOH prep
    • a vaginal fluid pH 4.5
    • a positive culture in the presence of symptoms

Treatment

Intravaginal agents

Butoconazole 2% cream 5 g intravaginally for 3 days,*†
Clotrimazole 1% cream 5 g intravaginally for 7-14 days,*†
Clotrimazole 100 mg vaginal tablet for 7 days,*
Clotrimazole 100 mg vaginal tablet, 2 tablets for 3 days,*
Clotrimazole 500 mg vaginal tablet, one tablet in a single application,*
Miconazole 2% cream 5 g intravaginally for 7 days,*†
Miconazole 200 mg vaginal suppository, one suppository for 3 days,*†
Miconazole 100 mg vaginal suppository, one suppository for 7 days,*†
Nystatin 100,000-unit vaginal tablet, one tablet for 14 days,
Ticonazole 6.5% ointment 5 g intravaginally in a single application,*†
Terconazole 0.4% cream 5 g intravaginally for 7 days,*
Terconazole 0.8% cream 5 g intravaginally for 3 days,*
Terconazole 80 mg vaginal suppository, one suppository for 3 days,*

Oral agent

Fluconazole 150 mg oral tablet, one tablet in a single dose

* These creams and suppositories are oil-based and might weaken latex condoms and diaphragms.
† OTC preparations

Pregnancy

• use only topical azole therapies
• most effective are butoconazole, clotrimazole, miconazole, terconazole
• 7 days of therapy recommended

Source: 1998 Guidelines for the Treatment of Sexually Transmitted Diseases. *MMWR.* 1997; 47: RR-1.

GYNECOLOGY

URINARY TRACT INFECTIONS

Fast Facts
- common symptoms are dysuria, frequency, and lower abdominal pain
- most common organisms
    - *E. coli*
    - *S. saprophyticus*
    - *Proteus mirabilis*
    - *Enterococcus sp.*
- ampicillin and tetracycline cause moniliasis in 25% of patients
- 50% resolve without therapy

Diagnosis
- UTI present if > 100,000 organisms on clean catch or >10,000 on cath specimen

Treatment
Non-pregnant
- single dose therapy (75-95%) effective
- consider other antibiotics depending on culture results

Pregnancy
- 5% of patients develop UTI or asymptomatic bacteriuria
- 1/3 untreated patients develop pyelonephritis
- pyelonephritis in pregnancy is treated as an inpatient
    - serum K^+ level on admission (may be hypokalemic)
- initiate renal evaluation for multiple admissions or left sided pyelonephritis
    - hydronephrosis usually occurs on the right because of uterine displacement
- consider suppression therapy for high risk patients

Regimen			
Pregnant Patients			
Nitrofurantoin	100 mg q 12 h x 7 d		
First-generation cephalosporin	500 mg q 6 h x 7 d		
Amoxicillin	500 mg q 8 h x 7 d		
Non-pregnant patients			
Single Dose		**7-Day**	
Nitrofurantoin	200 mg	TMP	100 (200) mg q 12 (24) h
Trimethoprim (TMP)	400 mg	TMP/sulfamethoxazole	160/800 mg q 12 h
TMP/sulfamethoxazole	300 mg / 1,600 mg	Nitrofurantoin	100 mg q 12 h
Amoxicillin	3 g	Amoxicillin	500 mg q 8 h
Ampicillin	3.5 g	First-generation cephalosporin	500 mg q 6 h
First-generation cephalosporin	2 g	Norfloxacin	400 mg q 12 h
Sulfisoxazole	2 g	Ofloxacin	200 mg q 12 h
		Ciprofloxacin	250 mg q 12 h
		Sulfisoxazole	500 mg q 6 h
		Tetracycline	500 mg q 6 h

Source: Management of Medical Disorders. *Primary and Preventive Care: A Primer for Obstetricians and Gynecologists.* American College of Obstetricians and Gynecologists, Washington, DC, 1994. Reproduced with permission.

PELVIC INFLAMMATORY DISEASE AND STDs
Fast Facts
- sequela of PID: adhesions, hydrosalpinx, 10x increase in ectopic, 4x increase in pelvic pain
- starts most often with cervical gonoccocal or *Chlamydia* leading to ascending infection
- 90% with lower abdominal pain
- 75% with mucopurulent cervical discharge
- 75% have ESR >15mm/hour
- 50% have WBC > 10,000 mm^3
- have low threshold to treat as inpatient

Diagnosis
All three should be present
1. History of lower abdominal pain and the presence of lower abdominal tenderness with or without evidence of rebound
2. Cervical motion tenderness
3. Adnexal tenderness (may be unilateral)

Additional criteria that support a diagnosis of PID include:
- oral temperature > 101°F (>38.3°C)
- abnormal cervical or vaginal discharge
- elevated erythrocyte sedimentation rate > 15 mm/hr
- elevated C-reactive protein
- laboratory documentation of cervical infection with *N. gonorrhoeae* or *C. trachomatis*

The definitive criteria for diagnosing PID in selected cases include:
- histopathologic evidence of endometritis on endometrial biopsy
- transvaginal ultrasonography or other imaging techniques showing thickened fluid-filled tubes with or without free pelvic fluid or tubo-ovarian complex, and
- laparoscopic abnormalities consistent with PID

Treatment
Outpatient
Regimen A
Ofloxacin, 400 mg PO bid for 14 days
    plus
Metronidazole, 500 mg PO bid for 14 days

Regimen B
Cefoxitin, 2 g IM plus probenecid 1 g orally in a single dose,
    or
Ceftriaxone, 250 mg IM or other parenteral third generation cephalosporin (e.g. cefotaxime or cefizoxime)
    plus
Doxycycline, 100 mg PO bid for 14 days

GYNECOLOGY

PELVIC INFLAMMATORY DISEASE AND STDs (CONT.)

Inpatient

Regimen A*

Cefoxitin, 2 g IV q6h, **or**

Cefotetan, 2 g IV q12h

   plus

Doxycycline, 100 mg PO or IV q12h

* The above regimen should be continued for at least 48 hours after the patient shows significant clinical improvement. After hospital discharge, doxycycline 100 mg PO bid should be continued for a total of 14 days.

Regimen B*

Clindamycin, 900 mg IV q8h

   plus

Gentamicin, loading dose IV or IM (2 mg/kg) followed by 1.5 mg/kg IV or IM q8h

* The above regimen should be continued for at least 48 hours after the patient shows significant clinical improvement. After hospital discharge, doxycycline 100 mg PO bid or clindamycin 450 mg PO qid should be continued for a total of 14 days.

Alternative Parenteral Regimens

Ofloxacin, 400 mg IV q12h *plus* metronidazole, 500 mg IV q8h

   OR

Ampicillin/Sulbactam, 3 g IV q6h *plus* doxycycline, 100 mg IV q12h

   OR

Ciprofloxacin, 200 mg IV q12h *plus* doxycycline, 100 mg PO q12h *plus* metronidazole, 500 mg IV q8h

Criteria for hospitalization

• Suspected pelvic or tubo-ovarian abscess
• Pregnancy (rare)
• Temperature > 38° C
• Uncertain diagnosis
• Nausea and vomiting precluding oral medications
• Upper peritoneal signs
• Failure to respond to oral antibiotics in 48 hr
• Noncompliant patient

Source: 1998 Guidelines for the Treatment of Sexually Transmitted Diseases. *MMWR.* 1997; 47: RR-1.

SEXUALLY TRANSMITTED DISEASES
Other Treatment Guidelines
Uncomplicated Gonoccocal Infections
A single dose of:
Ceftriaxone, 125 mg IM, or
Cefixime, 400 mg PO, or
Ciprofloxacin, 500 mg PO, or
Ofloxacin, 400 mg PO

     plus

A regimen effective against coinfection with *C. trachomatis,* such as doxycycline, 100 mg
PO bid for 7 days, or azithromycin, 1 g PO in a single dose.

Chlamydia
Recommended:
Doxycycline, 100 mg PO bid for 7 days, or
Azithromycin, 1 g orally in a single dose

Alternative:
Ofloxacin, 300 mg PO bid for 7 days, or
Erythromycin base, 500 mg PO qid for 7 days, or
Erythromycin ethylsuccinate, 800 mg PO qid for 7d, or
Sulfisoxazole, 500 mg PO qid for 10 days

Genital Herpes
Recommended regimens
Acyclovir, 400 mg PO tid for 7-10 days, or
Acyclovir, 200 mg PO 5 times/day for 7-10 days, or
Famciclovir, 250 mg PO tid for 7-10 days, or
Valacyclovir, 1 g PO bid for 7-10 days

Recommended regimen for episodic recurrent infection
Acyclovir, 400 mg PO tid for 5 days, or
Acyclovir, 200 mg PO 5 times/day for 5 days, or
Acyclovir, 800 mg PO bid for 5 days, or
Famciclovir, 125 mg PO tid for 5 days, or
Valacyclovir, 500 mg PO bid for 5 days

Recommended regimens for daily suppressive therapy
Acyclovir, 400 mg PO bid, or
Famciclovir, 250 mg PO tid, or
Valacyclovir, 250 mg PO bid, or
Valacyclovir, 500 mg PO once daily, or
Valacyclovir, 1,000 mg PO once daily

Source: 1998 Guidelines for the Treatment of Sexually Transmitted Diseases. *MMWR.* 1997; 47: RR-1.

GYNECOLOGY

SEXUALLY TRANSMITTED DISEASES (CONT.)

Syphilis

Patients with primary, secondary, or latent syphilis of < 1 years duration should receive:
Benzathine penicillin G, 2.4 million units IM in a single dose
Patients with latent syphilis of > 1 years duration or of unknown duration should receive:
Benzathine penicillin G 7.2 million units IM given as three weekly doses of 2.4 million units

External Genital Warts

Patient-applied:
Podofilox 0.5% solution or gel bid for 3 days followed by 4 days of no therapy. Repeat as needed x4. Total wart area <10 cm2, total volume podofilox <0.5 ml/day.
or

Imiquimod 5% cream; apply qhs three times/week for as long as 16 weeks

Provider-applied:
Cryotherapy
Podophyllin resin 10-25%
TCA or BCA 80-90%
Surgical removal

Chancroid

Recommended
Azithromycin, 1 g PO in a single dose, or
Ceftriaxone, 250 mg IM in a single dose, or
Erythromycin base 500 mg PO 4 times/day for 7 days, or
Ciprofloxacin 500 mg PO bid for 3 days

Source: 1998 Guidelines for the Treatment of Sexually Transmitted Diseases. *MMWR.* 1997; 47: RR-1.

ULCER-PRODUCING SEXUALLY TRANSMITTED DISEASES

Disease	Etiologic Agent	Characteristics of Ulcers	Specimen	Processing	Result
				Laboratory Diagnosis	
Syphilis Primary disease	Treponema pallidum	Ulcer typically singular, nontender, firm, with an erythematous base that is clean; the margins are raised, and the ulcer is painless. Nontreponemal tests: VDRL & RPR – 80% positive; Treponemal tests: FTA-ABS & MHA-TP – 85% positive	Serum from surface of chancre	Darkfield microscopy	Detection of T. pallidum
Syphilis Secondary disease	Treponema pallidum	Ulcers are usually multiple. Nontreponemal tests: 80% positive; Treponemal tests: 99% positive	Venous blood	Serum: FTA-ABS, MHA-TP, RPR, VDRL	Positive titer
Chancroid	Hemophilus ducreyi	Ulcer may be single or multiple, the lesion is well circumscribed, ulcer is irregular, base is erythematous, lesion is indurated and painful	Exudate from surface of ulcer	Gram's stain	Intracellular and extracellular bacteria, Gram-negative bacteria appear as "red school of fish"
Lymphogranuloma venereum	Chlamydia trachomatis	Serovars L1, L2 & L3. Ulcer is typically single; lesion usually has an erythematous base, clean margins, and is painless	Exudate from surface of ulcer	Culture or fluorescent antibody	Documentation of intracellular inclusions
Granuloma inguinal	Calymatobacterium granulomatis	Ulcer is usually multiple, dirty in appearance because of secondary infection, painless, unique characteristic: lesions appear as spreading ulcerating lesions	Exudate from surface, of ulcer	Gram's stain	Gram-negative bipolar organism resembles a safety pin
				Gemsia stain	Appear as encapsulated bacilli referred to as Donovan's bodies
Herpes simplex infection	Herpes simplex virus	Primary infection, multiple lesions, may vary in size from pinpoint to large; lesions usually have edema erythematous base but can become secondarily infected, thus producing a lesion that is covered in purulent exudate. Recurrent infection: characterized by 1 to 3 painful lesions	Aspirate of vesicular fluid or exudate from surface of ulcer	Culture	Cytoplasmic effect
				Fluorescent antibody, Tzanck cell test, Papanicolaou stain	Positive giant cells with inclusions

Source: Faro S and Stott G. Sexually transmitted diseases. *ObGyn Special Edition* 2001; 4:17-22. Reproduced with permission of the M-Mahon Publishing Group.

GYNECOLOGY

ECTOPIC PREGNANCY

Fast Facts
- incidence of ectopic pregnancy has increased since 1972, 108,000 ectopic pregnancies in 1992
- ectopic pregnancies represent 9% of all maternal deaths
- prior PID, especially related to *C. trachomatis*, is the major risk factor

Diagnosis
- serum β-hCG positive 8-9 days after ovulation
- β-hCG rises >66% in 48 hr with normal intrauterine pregnancy
  - β-hCG rises <66% in 48 hr in 15% of normal pregnancies
  - β-hCG rises >66% in 48 hr in 17% of ectopics
- Rule of 10's for normal pregnancies
  - β-hCG = 100 mIU/ml at time of missed menses
  - β-hCG = 100,000 mIU/ml at 10 weeks (peak)
  - β-hCG = 10,000 mIU/ml at term
- β-hCG elimination half-life = approximately 1 day
- 90% of ectopics have β-hCG < 6500 mIU/ml

Methotrexate Therapy
- reported success rates of 67-100% in selected patients

Absolute indications

Hemodynamically stable without active bleeding or signs of hemoperitoneum
Nonlaparoscopic diagnosis
Patient desires future fertility
General anesthesia poses a significant risk
Patient is able to return for follow-up care
Patient has no contraindications to methotrexate therapy

Relative Indications

Unruptured mass 3.5 cm at its greatest dimension
No fetal cardiac activity
β-hCG < 6500 mIU/ml (range 6,000-15,000 mIU/ml)

Absolute Contraindications

Breastfeeding
Overt or laboratory evidence of immunodeficiency
Alcoholism, alcoholic liver disease or other chronic liver disease
Preexisting blood dyscrasias, such as bone marrow hypoplasia, leukopenia, thrombocytopenia or anemia
Known sensitivity to methotrexate
Active pulmonary disease
Peptic ulcer disease
Hepatic, renal or hematologic dysfunction

Relative contraindications

Gestational sac 3.5 cm
Fetal cardiac activity

ECTOPIC PREGNANCY
Methotrexate Side Effects
Drug side effects
Nausea
Vomiting
Stomatitis
Diarrhea
Gastric distress
Dizziness
Severe neutropenia (rare)
Reversible alopecia (rare)
Pneumonitis

Treatment effects
Increase in abdominal pain in 2/3 of patients
Increase in β-hCG levels during first 1-3 days of treatment
Vaginal bleeding or spotting

Signs of treatment failure and tubal rupture
Significantly worsening abdominal pain, regardless of change in β-hCG levels
Hemodynamic instability
Levels of β-hCG that do not decline by at least 15% between day 4 and day 7 postinjection
Increasing or plateauing β-hCG levels after first week of treatment

Methotrxate Single Dose Protocol

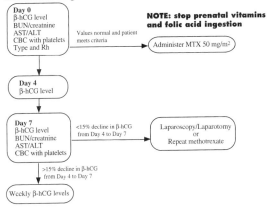

Day 0
β-hCG level
BUN/creatnine
AST/ALT
CBC with platelets
Type and Rh

Values normal and patient meets criteria

NOTE: stop prenatal vitamins and folic acid ingestion

Administer MTX 50 mg/m²

Day 4
β-hCG level

Day 7
β-hCG level
BUN/creatnine
AST/ALT
CBC with platelets

<15% decline in β-hCG from Day 4 to Day 7

Laparoscopy/Laparotomy
or
Repeat methotrexate

>15% decline in β-hCG from Day 4 to Day 7

Weekly β-hCG levels

GYNECOLOGY

ECTOPIC PREGNANCY - MANAGEMENT ALGORITHM

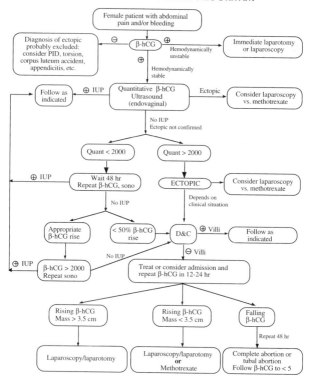

Adapted from Carson SA, Buster JE. Ectopic pregnancy. *N Engl J Med* 1993;329(16):1174-81, and Stovall TG, Ling FW. Ectopic pregnancy. Diagnostic and therapeutic algorithms minimizing surgical intervention. *J Reprod Med* 1993;38(10):807-12.

GYNECOLOGY

BODY SURFACE AREA NOMOGRAM

Height	Surface area	Weight
cm 200 — 79 in	2.80 m²	kg 150 — 330 lb

Height scale: cm 200–100, in 79–39

Surface area scale: 2.80 m² – 0.85 m²

Weight scale: kg 150 – 30, lb 330 – 66

Source: DiSaia PJ, Creasman WT. Epithelial ovarian cancer. In: *Clinical Gynecologic Oncology.* 4th ed. St. Louis: Mosby Year Book, 1993. Reproduced with the permission of the publisher.

GYNECOLOGY

EVALUATION OF THE SEXUAL ASSAULT PATIENT

Fast Facts
- sexual assault is the most underreported crime in the United States
- 50% of assaults occur in the victim's home
- Ob/Gyn physicians are often required to provide ER evaluation of rape victims
- use of special consent forms and rape victim evaluation kit can be helpful

Rape Tray Contents
1. Sealed package of microscope slides with frosted tips
2. Eye dropper bottle with 0.9% normal saline
3. Six to 12 packages of sterile cotton swabs
4. Eight to 12 sterile tubes
5. Urine container
6. Sterile, unused, and packaged comb
7. Sterile scissors
8. Two to four Pap smear mailers
9. Package of gummed labels
10. Nail scraper
11. An outline for conducting the examination

Evaluation
History
1. Age
2. Marital status
3. Parity
4. Menstrual history
5. Contraceptive usage
6. Time of last coitus prior to assault
7. Condom use at last coitus prior to assault and/or douching afterward
8. Drug or alcohol use
9. Past or present venereal disease
10. Mental illness or deficiency
11. Gynecologic surgery
12. Drug allergies
13. Description of the assailant and any knowledge of his identity
14. Circumstances surrounding the assault, particularly:
    - Did the assailant's penis penetrate the vulva?
    - Did the assailant experience orgasm?
    - Did the assailant wear a condom?
    - Did extragenital acts occur?
    - Did the assailant display or use a weapon?
15. Location of the assault
16. Time and date of the assault
17. Any reasons the assailant may have targeted the patient
18. Patient's actions since the assault, particularly:
    - douching
    - bathing or showering
    - urination
    - defecation
    - brushing teeth
    - changing clothes

142

EVALUATION OF THE SEXUAL ASSAULT PATIENT

Examination
• have patient disrobe while standing on white sheet
• place clothing in sealed plastic bag

  Pelvic Examination
  • note condition of pubic hair (? matted, bloody, etc.)
  • trauma to vulva
  • condition of hymen, anus, rectum
  • condition of vagina
  • condition of cervix

Laboratory Testing
• saline prep for sperm (note motility)
• Papanicolaou smear or Gram's stain for sperm (request on sheet)
• Gonorrhea and *Chlamydia* smear/culture (including rectal if appropriate)
• serologic testing for HIV, syphilis, Hepatitis B, CMV, HSV
• serum pregnancy test
• blood alcohol level, urine drug toxicology screen

Options for STD Prophylaxis
• 250 mg ceftriaxone IM plus 100 mg of doxycycline orally bid x 7 days
• 2 g spectinomycin IM plus 100 mg of doxycycline orally bid x 7 days
• 500 mg of erythromycin tid or 1 g of azithromycin (for pregnant patients)

Protection Against Pregnancy (Yuzpe Method)
• 2 doses taken 12 hours apart with an antiemetic (also see page 119)

Follow-up
• only 20-30% of patients will return for follow-up
• consider arranging for patient to be seen by same MD in follow-up

  Follow-up Testing
        2 weeks: Gonorrhea/*Chlamydia*
        4 weeks: Hepatitis B
        6 weeks: Pregnancy, Trichomonas, HPV, Vaginosis
        3 months: Gonorrhea/*Chlamydia*, HIV
        6 months: Hepatitis B, HIV, RPR

Source: Halbert, DR. Treating Rape Victims: Are You Prepared? *OBG Management*. 1995; 7(11): 39-50. Copyright 1995 Dowden Publishing Company, Montvale, NJ. Reproduced with permission.

GYNECOLOGY

PELVIC PAIN

Fast Facts

- frustrating disease for patient and physician
- many possible etiologies
- excessive use of narcotics can lead to drug dependancy

Etiology

Gynecologic

Extrauterine
- Adhesions
- Chronic ectopic pregnancy
- Chronic pelvic infection
- Endometriosis
- Residual ovary syndrome

Uterine
- Adenomyosis
- Chronic endometritis
- Leiomyomata
- Intrauterine contraceptive device
- Pelvic congestion
- Pelvic support defects
- Polyps

Urologic

- Chronic urinary tract infection
- Detrusor overactivity
- Interstitial cystitis
- Stone
- Suburethral diverticulitis
- Urethral syndrome

Gastrointestinal

- Cholelithiasis
- Chronic appendicitis
- Constipation
- Diverticular disease
- Enterocolitis
- Gastric/duodenal ulcer
- Inflammatory bowel disease (Crohns disease, ulcerative colitis)
- Irritable bowel syndrome
- Neoplasia

Musculoskeletal

- Coccydynia
- Disk problems
- Degenerative joint disease
- Fibromyositis
- Hernias
- Herpes zoster (shingles)
- Low back pain
- Levator ani syndrome (spasm of pelvic floor)
- Myofascial pain (trigger points, spasms)
- Nerve entrapment syndromes
- Osteoporosis (fractures)
- Pain posture
- Scoliosis/lordosis/kyphosis
- Strains/sprains

Other

- Abuse (physical or sexual, prior or current)
- Heavy metal poisoning (lead, mercury)
- Hyperparathyroidism
- Porphyria
- Psychiatric disorders (depression, bipolar disorders, inadequate personality disorder)
- Psychosocial stress (marital discord, work stress)
- Sickle cell disease
- Sleep disturbances
- Somatiform disorders
- Substance use (especially cocaine)
- Sympathetic dystrophy
- Tabes dorsalis (third-degree syphilis)

Source: American College of Obstetricians and Gynecologists. *Chronic Pelvic Pain*. ACOG Technical Bulletin, Number 223, May 1996. Copyright 1996 American College of Obstetricians and Gynecologists. Reproduced with permission.

PELVIC PAIN (CONT.)
Evaluation and Treatment Algorithm

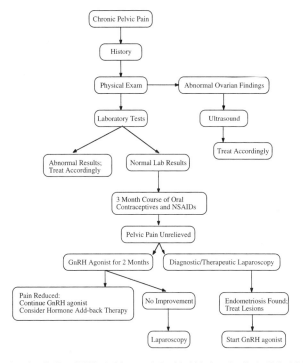

Chronic Pelvic Pain → History → Physical Exam → Laboratory Tests

Physical Exam → Abnormal Ovarian Findings → Ultrasound → Treat Accordingly

Laboratory Tests → Abnormal Results; Treat Accordingly

Laboratory Tests → Normal Lab Results → 3 Month Course of Oral Contraceptives and NSAIDs → Pelvic Pain Unrelieved

Pelvic Pain Unrelieved → GnRH Agonist for 2 Months / Diagnostic/Therapeutic Laparoscopy

GnRH Agonist for 2 Months → Pain Reduced: Continue GnRH agonist Consider Hormone Add-back Therapy

GnRH Agonist for 2 Months → No Improvement → Laparoscopy

Diagnostic/Therapeutic Laparoscopy → Endometriosis Found; Treat Lesions → Start GnRH agonist

Source: Carter, JE and Trotter, JP. GnRH analogs in the treatment of endometriosis: clinical and economic considerations. *The Female Patient* 1995; 20:13-18. Adapted with permission.

GYNECOLOGY

ENDOMETRIOSIS
Fast Facts
- found in 5-15% of reproductive age women undergoing laparoscopy
- 1/3 of these have infertility concerns
- CA 125 elevated in some cases
- symptoms: cyclic pre-and peri-menstrual pain, dyspareunia, chronic pelvic pain

Etiology
- Sampson: retrograde flow (monkey studies)
- Halban: lymphatic-vascular spreading (lung, brain, pericardium)
- Meyer: coelomic (found in males and infants)
- Dmowski: decrease in cellular immunity

Pathology
- ectopic endometrial glands
- ectopic endometrial stroma
- adjacent hemorrhage
- common locations: uterosacral ligament, ovary, cul-de-sac

Treatment
Medical
Primary therapy
GnRH agonists
- Buserelin
- Triptorelin
- Decapeptyl
- Goserelin (Zoladex)
- Leuprolide (Lupron)
- Nafarelin (Synarel)

Consider treatment of hypoestrogenic side effects
- daily medroxyprogesterone acetate 2.5 mg plus conjugated estrogens 0.625 mg
- daily norethindrone 1.0-5.0 mg daily

Alternatives (side effects, costs, duration of treatment >6 months)
Continuous oral contraceptives for 6-12 months
Medroxyprogesterone acetate 30 mg PO q day (must provide additional contraception)
Danazol 200-800 mg PO q day x 6 months

Surgical
Operative laparoscopy
- laser vs. electrocauterization for implants
Laparotomy for severe cases
Pain relief
- presacral neurectomy (midline pain)
- laparoscopic uterosacral nerve ablation (LUNA)
- consider post operative GnRH agonist therapy

GYNECOLOGY

GONADOTROPIN RELEASING HORMONE (GnRH) ANALOGS

Fast Facts
- native GnRH is a decapeptide
- substitutions at position 6 produce various agonists
- native LHRH isolated 1971 by Schally and Guillemin
- secreted in pulsatile fashion by hypothalamus
- serum half-life 2-8 minutes
- initiates synthesis and release of LH and FSH

Analogs
- most agonists substitution of D amino acid at position 6
- most antagonists substitutions and modification at position 2
- use of agonists results in transient upregulation of GnRH receptors followed by reversible downregulation and desensitization

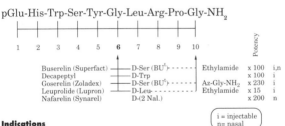

pGlu-His-Trp-Ser-Tyr-Gly-Leu-Arg-Pro-Gly-NH$_2$

		Potency	
Buserelin (Superfact)	D-Ser (BU^t) --- Ethylamide	x 100	i,n
Decapeptyl	D-Trp	x 100	i
Goserelin (Zoladex)	D-Ser (BU^t) --- Az-Gly-NH$_2$	x 230	i
Leuprolide (Lupron)	D-Leu --- Ethylamide	x 15	i
Nafarelin (Synarel)	D-(2 Nal.)	x 200	n

i = injectable
n = nasal

Indications
- endometriosis
- leiomyomata (preoperative shrinkage)
- IVF and other ART
- precocious puberty
- prostate carcinoma
- breast carcinoma (many trials)

Adverse Effects
- hypoestrogenic state (hot flashes, decreased libido, vaginal dryness, decreased bone mass)
- androgenic (acne, myalgias, edema, weight gain)

147

GYNECOLOGY

AMERICAN SOCIETY FOR REPRODUCTIVE MEDICINE SCORING SYSTEM FOR ENDOMETRIOSIS

AMERICAN SOCIETY FOR REPRODUCTIVE MEDICINE
REVISED CLASSIFICATION OF ENDOMETRIOSIS

Patient's Name _____ Date _____
Stage I (Minimal) - 1-5   Laparoscopy_____ Laparotomy_____ Photography_____
Stage II (Mild) - 6-15   Recommended Treatment_____
Stage III (Moderate) - 16-40
Stage IV (Severe) - >40
Total_____   Prognosis_____

PERITONEUM	ENDOMETRIOSIS		<1cm	1-3cm	>3cm
	Superficial		1	2	4
	Deep		2	4	6
OVARY	R	Superficial	1	2	4
		Deep	4	16	20
	L	Superficial	1	2	4
		Deep	4	16	20

	POSTERIOR CULDESAC OBLITERATION		Partial		Complete
			4		40

	ADHESIONS		<1/3 Enclosure	1/3-2/3 Enclosure	>2/3 Enclosure
OVARY	R	Filmy	1	2	4
		Dense	4	8	16
	L	Filmy	1	2	4
		Dense	4	8	16
TUBE	R	Filmy	1	2	4
		Dense	4*	8*	16
	L	Filmy	1	2	4
		Dense	4*	8*	16

*If the fimbriated end of the fallopian tube is completely enclosed, change the point assignment to 16.

Denote appearance of superficial implant types as red [(R), red, red-pink, flamelike, vesicular blobs, clear vesicles], white [(W), opacifications, peritoneal defects, yellow-brown], or black [(B) black, hemosiderin deposits, blue]. Denote percent of total described as R___%, W___% and B___%. Total should equal 100%.

Additional Endometriosis: _____   Associated Pathology: _____
_____   _____
_____   _____

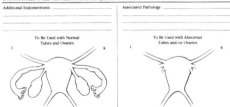

To Be Used with Normal Tubes and Ovaries   To Be Used with Abnormal Tubes and/or Ovaries

Source: Revised American Society for Reproductive Medicine classification of endometriosis: 1996. *Fertil. Steril.* 1997 (67):817-21. Reproduced with the permission of the publisher, the American Society for Reproductive Medicine.

EXAMPLES & GUIDELINES

STAGE I (MINIMAL)	STAGE II (MILD)	STAGE III (MODERATE)

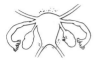

PERITONEUM
  Superficial Endo – 1-3cm – 2
R. OVARY
  Superficial Endo – < 1cm – 1
  Filmy Adhesions –/- < 1/3 – 1
                    TOTAL POINTS 4

PERITONEUM
  Deep Endo – > 3cm – 6
R. OVARY
  Superficial Endo – < 1cm – 1
  Filmy Adhesions –/- < 1/3 – 1
L. OVARY
  Superficial Endo – < 1cm – 1
                    TOTAL POINTS 9

PERITONEUM
  Deep Endo – > 3cm – 6
  CULDESAC
  Partial Obliteration – 4
L. OVARY
  Deep Endo – 1-3cm – 16
                    TOTAL POINTS 26

STAGE III (MODERATE)	STAGE IV (SEVERE)	STAGE IV (SEVERE)

PERITONEUM
  Superficial Endo – > 3cm – 4
R. TUBE
  Filmy Adhesions – < 1/3 – 1
R. OVARY
  Filmy Adhesions – < 1/3 – 1
L. TUBE
  Dense Adhesions – < 1/3 – 16*
L. OVARY
  Deep Endo – < 1cm – 4
  Dense Adhesions – < 1/3 – 4
                    TOTAL POINTS 30

PERITONEUM
  Superficial Endo – > 3cm – 4
L. OVARY
  Deep Endo – 1-3cm – 32**
  Dense Adhesions – < 1/3 – 8**
L. TUBE
  Dense Adhesions – < 1/3 – 8**
                    TOTAL POINTS 52

PERITONEUM
  Deep Endo – > 3cm – 6
  CULDESAC
  Complete Obliteration – 40
R. OVARY
  Deep Endo – 1-3cm – 16
  Dense Adhesions – < 1/3 – 4
L. OVARY
  Deep Endo – 1-3cm – 16
  Dense Adhesions – > 2/3 – 16
                    TOTAL POINTS 114

*Point assignment changed to 16
**Point assignment doubled

Determination of the stage or degree of endometrial involvement is based on a weighted point system. Distribution of points has been arbitrarily determined and may require further revision or refinement as knowledge of the disease increases.

To ensure complete evaluation, inspection of the pelvis in a clockwise or counterclockwise fashion is encouraged. Number, size and location of endometrial implants, plaques, endometriomas and/or adhesions are noted. For example, five separate 0.5cm superficial implants on the peritoneum (2.5 cm total) would be assigned 2 points. (The surface of the uterus should be considered peritoneum.) The severity of the endometriosis or adhesions should be assigned the highest score only for peritoneum, ovary, tube or culdesac. For example, a 4cm superficial and a 2cm deep implant of the peritoneum should be given a score of 6 (not 8.) A 4cm

deep endometrioma of the ovary associated with more than 3cm of superficial disease should be scored 20 (not 24.)

In those patients with only one adenexa, points applied to disease of the remaining tube and ovary should be multipled by two. **Points assigned may be circled and totaled. Aggregation of points indicates stage of disease (minimal, mild, moderate, or severe.)

The presence of endometriosis of the bowel, urinary tract, fallopian tube, vagina, cervix, skin etc., should be documented under "additional endometriosis." Other pathology such as tubal occlusion, leiomyomata, uterine anomaly, etc., should be documented under "associated pathology." All pathology should be depicted as specifically as possible on the sketch of pelvic organs, and means of observation (laparoscopy or laparotomy) should be noted.

Source: Revised American Society for Reproductive Medicine classification of endometriosis: 1996. *Fertil Steril.* 1997 (67):817-21. Reproduced with the permission of the publisher, the American Society for Reproductive Medicine.

GYNECOLOGY

LAPAROSCOPY
Fast Facts
- 1805 Bozzanie examines urethra with light reflector
- 1910 Jocobaeus in Sweden creates pneumoperitoneum in humans and uses endoscope
- 1968 Cohen and Fear write first American article in 30 years
- 1970's Semm in Germany describes techniques for adhesion lysis, adnexectomy and myomectomy
- 1972 American Association of Gynecologic Laparoscopists founded
- 1973 Shapiro and Adler describe laparoscopic removal of ectopic pregnancy

Indications
Diagnosis
- evaluation of benign pelvic mass
- pelvic pain
- acute (torsion, PID, ectopic, appendicitis, etc.)
- infertility
- evaluation of uterine perforation
- evaluation of pelvis prior to vaginal hysterectomy

Therapy
- sterilization
- fulguration of endometriosis
- ectopic pregnancy
- gamete intrafallopian transfer (GIFT)
- ovarian cystectomy
- oophorectomy
- lysis of adhesions
- appendectomy
- ? hysterectomy, myomectomy, incontinence surgery

Pre-op Evaluation
- patients must be well informed about all risks of planned procedure
- routine history and physical
- laboratory studies as indicated (ß-hCG, CBC, etc.)
- bowel prep where appropriate (GoLytely or Fleet's enema)
- antibiotics at discretion of surgeon

Critical Analysis
- fair evidence to suggest superiority of laparoscopy in treatment of:
  - ectopic pregnancy
  - endometriosis
  - PCOD resistant to clomiphene

Superiority of laparoscopy over laparotomy in more advanced procedures requires further evaluation and is more surgeon-specific.

150

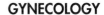

HYSTEROSCOPY

Fast Facts
- 1895 Bumm reports on uterine endoscope
- 1914 Heineberg introduces improved uteroscope
- 1925 Rubin describes using CO_2 as distension media
- 1968 Menken uses high viscosity media

Indications
Abnormal uterine bleeding
- diagnosis and therapy
  - ablation of endometrium
  - excision of endometrial polyps
  - excision of submucous fibroids

Intrauterine foreign bodies
- diagnosis and therapy
  - location of displaced IUD with visually directed removal of IUD
  - location of foreign bodies with visually directed removal of foreign bodies

Infertility or recurrent pregnancy wastage
- diagnosis and therapy
  - resection of müllerian fusion defects
  - division of endometrial adhesions

Distention Media

Distention Media	Advantages	Disadvantages	Complications
CO_2 gas	easy to operate; clear view	difficult if bleeding occurs	gas emboli
Low viscosity fluid (e.g., glycine, sorbitol)	easy to operate	mixing with blood causes image distortion	water intoxication hyponatremia/hypervolemia
High viscosity fluid (e.g., Dextran 70, Hyskon)	easy to operate; immiscible with blood	increased oncotic pressure, intravascular volume	anaphylactic shock noncardiogenic pulm. edema

Intrauterine evaluation

Anatomic Abnormality	Hysteroscopy	D&C	HSG	Ultrasound	MRI
Fibroids					
Intramural	+	-	+	+++	+++
Submucous	+++	+	++	++	+++
Intrauterine synechiae	+++	-	++	-	-
Bicornuate / septate uterus	+++	+	+++	+	+++
Endometrial polyps	++	+	+	+	++
Endometrial hyperplasia	+++	+++	-	+	-
Endometrial cancer	++	+++	+	+	-
Assessing tubal patency	+/-	-	+++	-	-

- not helpful; + ocasionally helpful; ++ often helpful; +++ very helpful

Sources: Corfman RS. Indications for hysteroscopy. *Obstet Gynecol Clin NA.* 1988;15(1):41-9. Reproduced with permission of the publisher W.B. Saunders Company. Lavy G. Hysteroscopy as a diagnostic aid. *Obstet Gynecol Clin NA.* 1988;15(1):61-72. Reproduced with permission of the publisher W.B. Saunders Company.

GYNECOLOGY

POST-OPERATIVE ORDERS:

1. Admit
2. Because... Diagnosis
3. Condition
4. Diet
5. Exercise... Activity
6. Fluids (IV)
7. Graphics (vitals, weights, urine output, etc.)
8. Hypersensitivities... Allergies
9. Input/Output
10. Junk (Foley, NG, SCD, spirometry, drains)
11. Call H.O. for...
12. Labs
13. Meds
14. Narcotics (see PCA orders)
15. O_2
16. Position (semi-Fowlers, knee chest, etc.)
17. Respiratory therapy
18. X-rays

Patient-Controlled Analgesia (PCA)

Drug	Bolus dose (mg)	Lockout Interval (min)	Continuous Infusion (mg/h)
Agonists			
Fentanyl	0.015-0.05	3-10	0.02-0.1
Hydromorphone	0.1-0.5	5-15	0.2-0.5
Meperidine	5-15	5-15	5-40
Methadone	0.5-3	10-20	
Morphine	0.5-3	5-20	1-10
Sufentanil	0.003-0.015	3-10	0.004-0.03
Agonists-Antagonists			
Buprenorphine	0.03-0.2	10-20	
Pentazocine	5-30	5-15	6-40

Typical PCA Orders

Morphine, 30 mg per 30 ml prefilled syringe
Loading dose=2 mg
Maintenance dose=1mg
Lockout interval=6 minutes
4 hour time limit at 20 mg
(if inadequate pain control increase to 30 mg)

Disregard all other opioid orders during PCA use.

Source: Management of Acute Postoperative Pain. In Barash PG, Cullen BF, Stoeling RK, eds. *Handbook of Clinical Anesthesia. 2nd edition.* Philadelphia: J.B. Lippincott, 1993. Reproduced with permission.

POST-OPERATIVE PAIN MANAGEMENT

Drug	Route	Maximum daily dose (mg)	Onset (h)	Peak (h)	Duration (h)
Nonopioids					
Salicylates					
Aspirin	PO	3,600	0.5-1	0-2	2-4
Diflunisal	PO	2,000	1-2	2-3	8-12
Propionic Acids					
Fenoprofen	PO	3,200	1	1-2	4-6
Ibuprofen	PO	3,200	0.5	1-2	4-6
Naproxen	PO	1,500	1	2-4	4-7
Indoles					
Indomethacin	PO	200	0.5	1-2	4-6
Sulindac	PO	400		2-4	
Ketorolac	IM	120	0.5-1	1	4-6
Oxicams					
Piroxicam	PO	20	1	3-5	48-72
p-Aminophenols					
Acetaminophen	PO	1,200	0.5	0.5-1	2-4
Phenacetin	PO	2,400		1	

Drug	Route	Dosage	Onset (h)	Peak (h)	Duration (h)
Opioids					
Morphine	IV	2.5	Rapid	0.125	
Codeine	IM	15-60	0.25-0.5	1-5	4-6
	PO	15-60	0.25-1	0.5-2	3-4
Hydromorphone	IM	1-4	0.3-0.5	1	2-3
Oxycodone	PO	5	0.5	1-2	3-6
Methadone	PO	2.5-10	05-1	1.5-2	4-8
Propoxyphene	PO	32-65	0.25-1	1-2	3-6
Meperidine	IM	0.3-0.6	0.12-0.5	1	2-4
Buprenorphine	IM	0.3-0.6	0.12	1	6-8
Butorphanol	IM	2-4	0.1-0.2	0.5-1	3-4
Nalbuphine	IM	10-20	0.25	1	3-6
	IV	1-5			
Pentazocine	IM	30-60	0.12-0.5	1-3	3-6
	PO	50			4-7

Source: Management of Acute Postoperative Pain. In Barash PG, Cullen BF, Stoeling RK, eds. *Handbook of Clinical Anesthesia. 2nd edition.* Philadelphia: J.B. Lippincott, 1993. Reproduced with permission.

GYNECOLOGY

SURGICAL RISKS IN PATIENTS WITH CARDIOVASCULAR DISORDERS

		Precautions
Atherosclerotic heart disease	Unstable angina Recent myocardial infarction Arrhythmias Congestive heart failure	Delay elective surgery 6 mo ECG and hemodynamic monitoring ECHO to assess LV function
Valvular heart disease	Endocarditis Congestive heart failure Critical aortic stenosis Anticoagulants	Antibiotic prophylaxis (see pg. 155) ECHO Hemodynamic monitoring
Congenital heart disease	Endocarditis (endarteritis) Thrombosis, hemorrhage	Antibiotic prophylaxis (see pg. 155) Evaluation of clotting status
Hypertension	Drug interactions	Maintenance of therapy for severe HTN only
Cardiomyopathy	Arrhythmias Congestive heart failure Anticoagulants	As for arteriosclerotic and valvular heart disease

Assessment of Risk of Venous Thrombosis

	Low Risk *	Moderate Risk ‡	High Risk ¥
Calf vein thrombosis	< 3%	10-30%	30-60%
Proximal vein thrombosis	< 1%	2-8%	6-12%
Pulmonary embolism	< 0.01%	0.1-0.7%	1-2%

* Under 40 years; operative procedure < 30 min; no immobilization
‡ Over 40 years; estrogen therapy; operative procedure > 30 min; obesity; post-operative infection
¥ Previous thromboembolism; abdominal or pelvic operation for malignant disease; immobilization

Source: Rock JA. Preoperative care. In: Thompson JD, Rock JA, Mattingly RF, Te Linde RW, ed. *Te Linde's Operative Gynecology*. 7th ed. Philadelphia: Lippincott, 1992, and from Bonnar J. Venous thromboembolism and gynecologic surgery. *Clin Obstet Gynecol*. 1985;28(2). Reproduced with the permission of the publishers.

Mitral Valve Prolapse

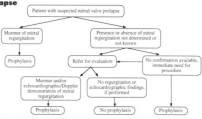

Source: Dajani AS, Taubert KA, Wilson W et al. Prevention of bacterial endocarditis: Recommendations by the American Heart Association. *JAMA*. 1997; 277(22):1794-1801. Reproduced with permission of the American Medical Association.

154

BACTERIAL ENDOCARDITIS PROPHYLAXIS

Indications for Prophylaxis

Negligible-risk category (no greater risk than the general population)

Isolated secundum atrial septal defect
Surgical repair of atrial septal defect, ventricular septal defect, or patent ductus arteriosus
(without residua beyond 6 mo.)
Previous coronary artery bypass graft surgery
Mitral valve prolapse without valvar regurgitation
Physiologic, functional, or innocent heart murmurs
Previous Kawasaki disease without valvar dysfunction
Previous rheumatic fever without valvar dysfunction
Cardiac pacemakers (intravascular and epicardial) and implanted defibrillators

Moderate-risk category

Most other congenital cardiac malformations (other than listed here)
Acquired valvar dysfunction (e.g., rheumatic heart disease)
Hypertrophic cardiomyopathy
Mitral valve prolapse with valvar regurgitation and/or thickened leaflets

High-risk category

Prosthetic cardiac valves, including bioprosthetic and homograft valves
Previous bacterial endocarditis
Complex cyanotic congenital heart disease
(eg, single ventricle states, transposition of the great arteries, tetralogy of Fallot)
Surgically constructed systemic pulmonary shunts or conduits

Recommended: Surgical operations involving intestinal mucosa; cystoscopy; urethral dilation
NOT Recommended: Vaginal hysterectomy*; vaginal delivery*; Cesarean section; In uninfected tissue: urethral catheterization; uterine dilation and curettage; therapeutic abortion; sterilization procedures; insertion/removal of IUD
* Treatment optional in high-risk patients.

Antibiotics and Dosage

SBE Prophylaxis

High-risk patients

Ampicillin 2.0 g intramuscularly (IM) or intravenously (IV) plus gentamicin 1.5 mg/kg (not to exceed 120 mg) within 30 minutes of starting the procedure; 6 hr later, ampicillin 1 g IM/IV or amoxicillin 1 g orally

High-risk patients allergic to ampicillin/amoxicillin

Vancomycin 1.0 g IV over 1-2 hr plus gentamicin 1.5 mg/kg IV/IM (not to exceed 120 mg); complete injection infusion within 30 minutes of starting the procedure

Moderate-risk patients

Amoxicillin 2.0 g orally 1 hr before procedure, or ampicillin 2.0 g IM/IV within 30 minutes of starting the procedure

Moderate-risk patients allergic to ampicillin/amoxicillin

Vancomycin 1.0 g IV over 1-2 hr; complete infusion within 30 minutes of starting the procedure

Source: Dajani AS, Taubert KA, Wilson W et al. Prevention of bacterial endocarditis: Recommendations by the American Heart Association. *JAMA.* 1997; 277(22):1794-1801. Reproduced with permission of the American Medical Association.

GYNECOLOGY

UROGYNECOLOGY

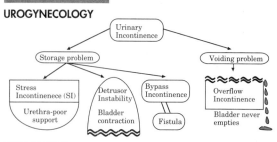

Stress Incontinence

Definition: Loss of urine in absence of bladder contraction
Pathology: Poor support of bladder base
Evaluation:
1) History
   • loss of urine with cough or sneeze (reliable in 75%)
2) Physical examination
   • presence of cystocele
   • neurologic assessment
      • sensation (S2-4) inner thighs, perirectal, vulvar
      • bulbocavernous motor reflex (gentle touch to clitoris)
3) Q-tip test
   • place cotton swab to bladder, patient pushes while supine
   • angle change of >35° suggestive of poor urethrovesicle support
4) Cystometry
   • fill bladder to capacity while measuring pressures
   • normal bladder (SI patients) has no contractions while filling
Treatment:
1) Surgery (always have pre-op cystometrics)
   • Anterior colporrhaphy and Kelly plication (+ 75% cure rate)
   • Needle suspension procedures (~ 80% cure rate, requires cystoscopy)
      • Stamey, modified Pereyra, Raz
   • Abdominal retropubic suspension (85-90% cure rate)
      • Marshal-Marchetti-Kranz, Burch
   • Periurethral collagen injections (previous failures, office procedure)

2) Non-Surgical modalities
   • Estrogen vaginal cream for 6 weeks (good result in 40%)
   • α-sympathomimetics (affects periurethral smooth muscle ~ 30%)
   • Kegel exercise (periurethral striated muscles ~ 40%)
   • Electrical stimulation ("passive" Kegel, stimulated pudendal ~ 40%)
   • Vaginal pessary (supports bladder base - good result in 40%)

Detrusor Instability

Definition: Appearance of contraction (> 15 cm of water) when filling bladder

Pathology: Idiopathic in 85%, neuropathy (detrusor dysnergia) in 15%

Evaluation:

1) History: urinary urgency, frequency and nocturia (50% reliable)
2) Physical exam: rule out neuropathy, see "stress incontinence"
3) Cystometry: appearance of bladder contraction during filling

Treatment:

1) Medications
   - Tolterodine tartrate (Detrol LA) 4 mg PO daily
   - Oxybutynin (Ditropan) 5 mg PO tid
   - Propantheline bromide (Pro-banthine) 15 mg PO tid
   - Imipramine (Tofranil) 50 mg PO tid
2) Behavior modification: timed voiding
3) Electrical stimulation: similar to stress incontinence

Bypass Incontinence

Definition: Loss of urine at all times

Pathology: Fistula: vesicovaginal, urethrovaginal, ureterovaginal

Etiology: Pelvic surgery, cancer (radiation therapy), obstetrical trauma

Evaluation:

1) History: continuous leakage
2) Physical exam: spill of dye from bladder (catheter or IV)

Treatment:

1) Surgical repair
   - simple vaginal repair (Lazko procedure)
   - abdominal approach in complicated situations
   - urinary diversion (usually in cancer patients)

Overflow Incontinence

Definition: Incomplete voiding with overflow of urine from distended bladder

Pathology: Hypotonic bladder (medications, surgery), spastic or scarred urethra

Etiology: Pelvic surgery, medication, psychogenic

Evaluation:

1) History: urgency, frequency, nocturia, frequent UTI's
2) Physical exam: neurologic assessment
3) Cystourethroscopy: assess condition of urethra, check post-void residual
4) Urodynamics: hypotonicity of bladder versus spasticity of urethra

Treatment:

1) Scarred urethra
   - surgery
   - urethral dilation
2) Spastic urethra
   - Diazepam (Valium)
   - Phenoxybenzaline (Dibenzilin)
3) Hypotonic bladder
   - Bethenechol (Urecholin)

Courtesy of A. Bergman, M.D., Department of Obstetrics and Gynecology, University of Southern California

GYNECOLOGY

VULVAR DYSTROPHIES
Non-neoplastic epithelial disorders
• new classification based on gross and histopathologic findings

I. Squamous cell hyperplasia (formerly hyperplastic dystrophy)
II. Lichen sclerosus
III. Other dermatoses

Squamous cell hyperplasia
• most represent lichen simplex chronicus
• gross appearance variable
• microscopic evaluation
    • hyperkeratosis
    • acanthosis
    • parakeratosis

Lichen sclerosus
• classic lesion - crinkled (cigarette paper), parchment-like
• biopsy
    • hyperkeratosis
    • epithelial thinning

• often associated with foci of hyperplastic and thinning epithelium ("mixed dystrophy")
    • squamous cell hyperplasia found in 27-35%
    • intraepithelial neoplasia found in 5%

Therapy
• biopsy, biopsy, biopsy

Squamous cell hyperplasia
• topical steroids (bid to tid)
• 0.025-0.01% triamcinolone acetonide
• 0.1% β-methasone valerate and crotamiton (Eurax) in 7:3 mix

Lichen sclerosus
• topical testosterone no longer recommended
• clobetasol (Temovate 0.05%) cream very effective
    • use bid x 1 month, then q hs x 2 months, then 2x/week for 3 months
        • complete regression can occur with this treatment
• crotamiton (Eurax) 10% cream for pruritus

Adapted from American College of Obstetricians and Gynecologists. *Vulvar Dystrophies*. Technical Bulletin 139, January 1990.

HORMONE REPLACEMENT THERAPY CHOICES

Active Ingredients	Drug Name	Company	Typical Daily Dosage Choices
Estrogens			
Conjugated equine estrogens (CEE)	Premarin	Wyeth-Ayerst	0.3, 0.625, 0.9, 1.25, 2.5 mg/continuous daily dosing or cyclic dosing
17-β estradiol (oral)	Estrace	Warner Chilcott	0.5, 1, 2 mg/continuous daily dosing
17-β estradiol (transdermal)	Climara	Berlex	0.025, 0.05, 0.075, 0.1 mg weekly patch
	Alora	Watson	0.05, 0.075, 0.1 mg/change patch 2x/wk
	Esclim	Women First	0.025, 0.0375, 0.05, 0.075, 0.1 mg/change patch 2x/wk
	Estraderm	Novartis	0.05, 0.1 mg/change patch 2x/wk
	Vivelle-dot	Novartis	0.0375, 0.05, 0.075, 0.1 mg/change patch 2x/wk
Estropipate	Ogen	Pharmacia	0.625, 1.25, 2.5 mg/continuous daily dosing or cyclic dosing
	Ortho-EST	Women First	0.625, 1.25 mg/continuous daily dosing or cyclic dosing
Esterified estrogens	Estratab	Solvay	0.3, 0.625, 1.25, 2.5 mg/continuous daily dosing
	Menest	Monarch	0.3, 0.625, 1.25, 2.5 mg/cyclic dosing (3 wk on therapy, 1 wk off)
Synthetic conjugated estrogens	Cenestin	Duramed/Solvay	0.625, 0.9, 1.25 mg/continuous daily dosing
Oral Estrogen-Progestin Combination Therapy			
Conjugated equine estrogens and medroxyprogesterone acetate (MPA)	PremPro	Wyeth-Ayerst	0.625 mg CEE plus 2.5 mg MPA, 0.625 mg CEE plus 5 mg MPA
	PremPhase	Wyeth-Ayerst	0.625 mg CEE days 1-14, 0.625 mg CEE plus 5 mg MPA days 15-28
Ethinyl estradiol (EE) and norethindrone acetate (NE)	Fem HRT	Parke-Davis	5 mcg EE plus 1 mg NE: continous daily dosing
Micronized estradiol and norgestimate	Ortho-Prefest	Ortho-McNeil	1 mg 17-β estradiol (continous) and 0.09 mg norgestimate (pulsed in 3-day cycles)
Micronized estradiol and norethindrone acetate (NE)	Activella	Pharmacia	1 mg 17-β estradiol and 0.5 mg NE: continuous daily dosing
Combination Oral Estrogen and Testosterone			
Conjugated equine estrogens and methyltestosterone (MT)	Estratest	Solvay	1.25 mg CEE plus 2.5 mg MT: cyclic dosing (3 wk on therapy, 1 wk off)
	Estratest-HS		0.625 mg CEE plus 1.25 mg MT: cyclic dosing (3 wk on therapy, 1 wk off)
Transdermal Combination Therapy			
17-β estradiol and norethindrone acetate (NE)	CombiPatch	Aventis	0.05 mg 17-β estradiol and 0.14 mg NE or 0.05 mg 17-β estradiol and 0.25 mg NE, change patch 2x/wk
Vaginal Estrogen Therapy			
Conjugated equine estrogens	Premarin	Wyeth-Ayerst	0.625 mg/gram; daily
17-β estradiol	Estrace	Warner Chilcott	0.1 mg/gram; daily then 1-3x/wk
Estropipate	Ogen	Pharmacia	1.5 mg/gram; daily
Dienestrol	Ortho Dienestrol	Ortho-McNeil	0.1 mg/gram; daily then 1-3x/wk
Estradiol	Vagifem	Pharmacia	25 mg tablets daily for 2 weeks then 2x/wk
Vaginal Estrogen Ring			
Estradiol	Estring	Pharmacia	2 mg reservoir, replace every 90 days

MENOPAUSE

HRT OPTIONS

Cyclical Sequential
• earliest form of combined HRT but is confusing for the patient to take
• results in several days a month without estrogen.

Continuous Sequential ("cyclical")
• perimenopausal women are often started on continuous sequential HRT and then switched over to continuous combined HRT after a few years when the ovary is less likely to intermittently function and cause breakthrough bleeding.

Continuous Combined ("continuous")
• perimenopausal women are often started on continuous sequential HRT and then switched over to continuous combined HRT after a few years when the ovary is less likely to intermittently function and cause breakthrough bleeding.

Cyclical Combined
• good record in achieving amenorrhea within 9 months (>90%)
• estrogen can be given for 25 days or for the full 30 days a month depending on symptoms during the pill free days.

3 Day Cyclic On-off Regimen
• allows the estrogen and progesterone receptors to up-regulate, reducing progestin needed and minimizing the progestin-related side effects

Long cyclic HRT
• unacceptable high risk for endometrial hyperplasia and cancer.

Estrogen

Progestin

COMMON HRT PROBLEMS

Solutions for Common HRT Problems	Additional Options
PMS symptoms	
Increase exercise. Vitamin B6 50-100 mg daily. Decrease salt/sugar intake.	Change to low dose oral contraceptive. Change to low dose patch (e.g. Climara 0.025mg) weekly during the progestin phase and extend into the menstrual week. Withdrawal bleeding will still occur. Consider using oral micronized progesterone 100-200 mg qhs during progestin phase (has sedative and anxiolytic properties). Consider Maxzide 25 mg qd for mild diuresis.
Breast tenderness	
Restart HRT at lower estrogen dose and increase slowly.	Change HRT to a patch for steadier levels. Change progestin to norethindrone or oral micronized progesterone. Add methyltestosterone (e.g. HS Estratest).
Hot flashes	
Double estrogen dosage for 3-6 months then taper or change estrogen to a patch for steadier levels or add testosterone.	
Insomnia	
Recommend patient take estrogen in AM (stimulant) and to change the progestin to oral micronized progesterone at bedtime (sedative).	
Vaginal dryness	
Apply 1/2 applicator of estrogen cream PV 2-3x weekly at bedtime or use the Estring vaginal ring (3 months).	
Breakthrough bleeding	
Consider endometrial biopsy if >35 years Change to cyclical combined or continuous sequential (see diagram).	Consider a progesterone IUD. Perform hysteroscopy and D&C.
Breast cancer anxiety	
Provide appropriate counseling. Consider using a lower dose of estrogen (e.g 0.3 mg CEE or 0.5 mg estradiol) or use raloxifene.	

MENOPAUSE

OSTEOPOROSIS

Fast Facts
- ~15% of all Caucasian post-menopausal women are affected
- ~50% of Causasian women will experience an osteoporotic fracture in her lifespan
- 1995 cost for osteoporotic fractures was $14 billion

Recommendations to the Physician
- Advise patients to quit smoking, decrease alcohol intake and start weight-bearing exercise
- Advise patients to obtain the needed amount of calcium and 400-800 IU vitamin D per day
- Perform bone mineral density (BMD) testing on appropriate patients (see below)

Recommended Daily Calcium Intake

Young adults/pregnant and lactating women	1,200 mg per day
Premenopausal women	1,000 mg per day
50-64 and on HRT	1,000 mg per day
50-64 and not on HRT	1,500 mg per day
65 yrs	1,500 mg per day

Calcium Supplementation

Product (% elemental Ca^{2+})		Total weight (mg)	Total elemental Ca^{2+} (mg)
Calcium carbonate (40%)	Os-Cal 500	1,250	500
	Tums	500	200
	Titralac	420	168
Calcium citrate (21.2%)	Citrical 950	950	200
Calcium lactate (13%)	Generic	325	42.2
Calcium phosphate (38%)	Posture	1,565	600

Osteoporosis Testing
DEXA (dual x-ray beam at hip and spine)
- most commonly used method to test BMD
- T Score
  - the amount of standard deviations compared to a young and normal adult of the same sex

0 to -1	Normal
-1 to -2.5	Osteopenia
< -2.5	Osteoporosis
< -2.5 with fragility fractures	Severe osteoporosis

Testing for BMD
- all women > 65 years of age
- all post-menopausal women with a newly diagnosed fracture
- all post-menopausal women less than 65 years who have one or more risk factors, besides menopause, for osteoporotic fractures

162

OSTEOPOROSIS

Risk factors

Non-modifiable
- personal history of fracture as an adult
- history of adult fracture in first degree relatives
- Caucasian race
- advanced age
- dementia
- poor health/frailty

Potentially Modifiable
- current cigarette smoking
- low body weight (<127 lbs)
- low lifelong calcium intake
- estrogen deficiency (early menopause <45 y/o or prolonged (>1 yr) premenopausal amenorrhea)
- impaired eyesight despite adequate correction
- recurrent falls
- inadequate physical health

Treatment

All women who have osteoporosis per BMD testing should be treated primarily with HRT or bisphophonates since they are the most effective. If the BMD testing shows osteopenia, treatment for osteoporosis prevention can also be offered. If bisphophonates are used for osteoporosis prevention, half the normal dose should be used.

Medical treatment of osteoporosis

Agents	Dosage	Comments
Estrogen	0.625 mg CEE or Estradiol 1mg	Greatest benefit relative to cost Reduces new fractures by 50% Bone density drops rapidly after HRT discontinued
Alendronate (Fosamax)	Prevention 5 mg daily or 35 mg weekly Treatment 10mg daily or 70 mg weekly	Take with 6-8 oz. water Do not eat or drink for the following 30 minutes Do not lie down for at least 30 minutes Reduces new fractures by 50% 10 yr half life, so no rapid drop in bone density after stopping drug
Risedronate (Actonel)	Prevention and treatment 5 mg daily	Take with 6-8 oz. water Do not eat or drink for the following 30 minutes Do not lie down for at least 30 minutes Reduces new fractures by 50% 10 yr half life, so no rapid drop in bone density after stopping drug
Calcitonin Nasal Spray (Miacalcin)	200 IU/d (1 spray)	Alternate nostrils daily Can be taken at any time Has bone analgesic qualities Reduces new fractures by 30%
Raloxifene (Evista)	Prevention 60 mg daily	Can be taken at any time Reduces new fractures by 30%

MENOPAUSE

OSTEOPOROSIS THERAPY

Agent	Mechanism of Action	Effect on Bone	Effect on Fractures	Recommended for:	Risks	Comments
Calcium	Increased availability	Deficiency causes loss; supplements reduce loss	Reduction in fracture risk by use of calcium with vitamin D	Adolescents, lactating women, hypoestrogenic women, osteoporosis risk factors including age	Should not exceed 2,000 mg daily; hypercalcuria, hypercalcemia	Revised daily requirement
Vitamin D	Increased intestinal absorption of calcium	Direct effect unknown; increases bone mass when combined with calcium	Reduction in fracture risk by use of calcium with vitamin D	Institutionalized elderly and women over 70	Hypercalcuria and hypercalcemia with increased doses	Overdose in elderly can lead to renal failure
Estrogen	Reduces bone resorption by inhibiting osteoclasts	Slows bone loss, increases bone mass slightly; affects all types of bone	Documented reduction of all fractures; as high as 50% reduction of hip fractures	First-line choice for prevention in absence of contraindications; indicated for proven osteoporosis or abnormal bone density	Uterine bleeding, endometrial hyperplasia, endometrial cancer	Additional cardiovascular and other benefits have been described
Alendronate	Reduces bone resorption by inhibiting osteoclasts	Slows bone loss, increases bone mass	Significant reduction (48%) in new vertebral fractures	Treatment of osteoporosis (10 mg dose); prevention of repeat vertebral fractures	Not recommended for patients with renal insufficiency or upper gastrointestinal problems	Use as a preventative in normal population (5 mg dose)

Source: American College of Obstetricians and Gynecologists. Osteoporosis. *ACOG Educational Bulletin*, 1998; Number 246. Reproduced with permission.

OSTEOPOROSIS THERAPY (CONT)

Agent	Mechanism of Action	Effect on Bone	Effect on Fractures	Recommended for:	Risks	Comments
Calcitonin	Reduces bone resorption by inhibiting osteoclasts	Increases vertebral bone mass	Significant reduction in new vertebral fractures	Alternative to estrogen therapy	Development of neutralizing antibodies – effect unknown	Objection to injections now avoided by intranasal spray; absorption is variable
Raloxifene	Reduces bone resorption by inhibiting osteoclasts	Slight increase in bone mass over 2-3 years		Prevention of osteoporosis		Low rate of uterine bleeding
Progestins	Reduces bone resorption by inhibiting osteoclasts	Slows bone loss	Long-term study of progestins alone unavailable	Women on estrogen replacement therapy unless uterus surgically absent; not recommended as sole agent	Dosage required to positively affect bone causes reduction in HDL and increases in LDL	
Fluoride	Deposited and concentrated in bone; slowly reabsorbed	Increases bone mass in continuous manner; new bone is structurally abnormal	No demonstrated reduction in vertebral fractures; may increase non-vertebral fractures	Not recommended in United States	New bone may be weaker and increase fracture risk	Slow-release formulations may improve effectiveness of fluoride
Etidronate	Inhibits bone resorption by reducing ability of osteoclasts to resorb bone	Increases bone mass, reduces bone remodeling	Reduction not clearly demonstrated	Not FDA approved for this purpose	Inhibits mineralization at slightly higher doses; long-term effects unknown	Approved for osteoporosis treatment in Canada
Tamoxifen	Assumed to be an anti-absorptive agent with an effect of a weak estrogen	Laboratory evidence of reduced bone loss in rats	No long-term data	Not recommended as an agent specific for osteoporosis prevention	Endometrial carcinoma incidence is reportedly increased	Level of protection against osteoporosis unknown; other agents should be added

Source: American College of Obstetricians and Gynecologists. Osteoporosis. *ACOG Educational Bulletin*. 1998; Number 246. Reproduced with permission.

NON-MALIGNANT CONDITIONS OF THE BREAST

Disease State	Etiology	Pathophysiology	Clinical Presentation
Fat necrosis	Trauma, ischemia	Degenerating adipocytes free fatty acids and elicit inflammatory response.	Often mobile, firm, occasionally with induration, frequent history of antecedent trauma.
Cystic duct dilation	Progesterone stimulation of estrogen primed ducts Duct obstruction (scarring, intraductal hyperplasia)	Stimulation of secretion leads to duct dilation. Obstruction of ducts leads to retrograde dilation and inspissation of secretions. Extravasated cyst fluid may cause intense inflammatory reaction. Various pharmacologic agents.	Pliant to fluctuant mass, usually in complexes; if deep, may be firm; often varies with menstrual cycle; most prominent in luteal phase; occasionally accompanied by nipple discharge.
Fibroadenoma	Estrogen stimulation at onset of puberty and at time of corpus luteum failure during perimenopausal and anovulatory cycles	Proliferation of fibrous tissue, possibly secondary to unopposed estrogen stimulation.	Usually small, unilateral, firm but resilient mass, freely movable and slow growing; may show cystic changes; most common tumor in menstruating women after age 25.
Mastitis	Extravasated or inspissated secretions Infection	Inflammatory reaction to cyst fluid from dilated alveoli, duct ectasia secondary to infection (usually *S. aureus*).	Acute or chronic mastodynia; often bilateral, with tenderness, redness; infective mastitis may respond to broad spectrum antibiotics.
Sclerosing adenosis	Unknown	Myoepithelial proliferation disrupts typical alveolar formation, producing an infiltrative pattern of parenchymal cells.	Occasionally a firm, fixed mass that may mimic cancer but is usually not a distinct mass.
Hyperplasia of lobules	Excessive or prolonged exposure to estrogenic stimuli	Excessive estrogen stimulation; various pharmacologic agents.	May be associated with galactorrhea and focal lactational change; usually found incidental to other palpable pathology.
Intraductal acinar epithelial hyperplasia	Hormonal	Estrogen stimulation in absence of progesterone may cause epithelial proliferation; early proliferative change varies with menstrual cycle; more severe forms may be hormonally unresponsive; severe hyperplasias with atypia strongly associated with cancer.	Papillomatosis may be suspected due to bloody nipple discharge; hyperplasia is usually found incidentally, in biopsy obtained to explain other clinically apparent changes.
Duct ectasia	Obstruction, atrophy; possibly inverted nipples; lactation	Distension of terminal collecting ducts, intense periductal inflammation due to extravasated secretions.	Nipple discharge or retraction may occur if scarring is extensive.

Source: Shingleton WW, McCarty KS. What you should know about breast pathology. *Cont Ob/Gyn* 1987;29(2):90. Reproduced with the permission of the publisher Medical Economics Publishing, Montvale, NJ.

BREAST DISEASE

FINE NEEDLE ASPIRATION OF A BREAST CYST

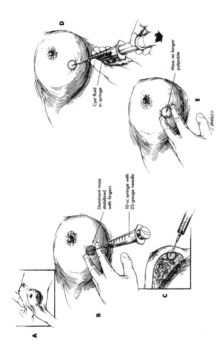

(A) The mass is palpated, and the skin is wiped with an alcohol sponge. (B, C) The needle penetrates the cyst without passing through the opposite wall. No local anesthesia is necessary. (D, E) Fluid is withdrawn until the mass disappears.

Source: Nichols DH. *Gynecologic and Obstetric Surgery.* Chicago: Mosby Year Book, 1993. Reproduced with the permission of the publisher.

BREAST DISEASE

FINE NEEDLE ASPIRATION OF A BREAST LUMP

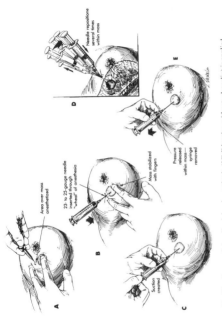

(A) After the mass is localized, local anesthesia (1% lidocaine without adrenalin) is applied. (B) The mass is stabilized, and the needle inserted. (C) Suction is created as the needle is withdrawn. (D) The needle is repositioned several times. (E) Suction is released as the needle is withdrawn.

Source: Nichols DH. *Gynecologic and Obstetric Surgery.* Chicago: Mosby Year Book, 1993. Reproduced with the permission of the publisher.

BREAST DISEASE

BREAST CANCER

Fast Facts
- leading site of cancer in women (see page 183) with a 12.6% lifetime risk
- leading cause of death from cancer in women 35-54 years old
- risk of death from breast cancer has remained constant at 3.6%
  - more than 80% of patients live longer than 5 years
- 80% of women with breast cancer have no known risk factor

Risk Factors

Family History

First degree relative with breast cancer	x 1.8
Premenopausal first-degree relative with breast cancer	x 3.0
Premenopausal first-degree relative with bilateral breast cancer	x 9.0
Postmenopausal first-degree relative with breast cancer	x 1.5
Postmenopausal first-degree relative with bilateral breast cancer	x 3.5

Ovarian function

Oophorectomy before age 35	x 0.4
Anovulatory menstrual cycles	x 2.0 to x 4.0

Age at menopause

Before age 45	x 0.5 to x 0.7
Age 45-54	x 1.0
After age 55	x 1.5
After age 55 with > 40 menstrual years	x 2.5 to 5.0

Nutritional

Obesity, diabetes, high-fat diet	x 1.0 to 4.0

Pregnancy

Before age 20	x 0.4
First child age 20-34	x 1.0
First child at > age 35	x 1.5 to x 4.0
Nulliparous	x 1.3 to x 4.0

Fibrocystic condition

Duct ectasia	x 1.0
Sclerosing adenosis	x 1.0
Blunt duct adenosis	x 1.0
Fibroadenoma	x 1.0
Cystic disease without hyperplasia	x 1.2
Ductor or intra-acinar epithelial hyperplasia	x 2.8 to x 6.0
Atypical lobular hyperplasia (ALH)	x 4.0
ALH < 45 years old	x 3.9
ALH > 45 years old	x 6.0
Lobular carcinoma in situ (LCIS)	x 12.0
Ipsilateral breast	x 18.0
Contra lateral breast	x 9.0

Source: Shingleton WW, McCarty KS. What you should know about breast pathology. *Cont Ob/Gyn* 1987;29(2):90. Reproduced with the permission of the publisher Medical Economics Publishing, Montvale, NJ.

BREAST CANCER (CONT.)

Biopsy Indications
- cyst aspiration and fine needle aspiration are crucial in clinical evaluation of breast disease
- perform open biopsy if one of the following is present:
  - equivocal findings on aspiration
  - bloody cyst fluid
  - recurrence of cyst after 1-2 aspirations
  - bloody nipple discharge
  - nipple excoriation
  - skin edema or erythema suspicious of inflammatory breast carcinoma

Management
- follow-up, follow-up, follow-up
- mammography alone is not sufficient in palpable breast lump
- listen to the patient
- see open biopsy indications
- choice of surgical therapy dependent on several factors

Prognosis
- axillary node status is most important prognostic feature
- higher recurrence rates in E2 receptor negative tumors
- DNA ploidy studies also predictive (aneuploid worse)

Breast Cancer and Pregnancy
- 2% of cancers diagnosed in pregnancy
- pregnancy delays diagnosis, but no effect on prognosis
- 1st trimester
  - mastectomy/axillary nodes
  - wide local excision and radiation contraindicated
  - TAB does not improve survival
- 2nd trimester
  - as above
- 3rd trimester
  - depends on maturity
  - consider observation until delivery
- chemotherapy probably safe in 2nd, 3rd trimester

Mammography Guidelines (controversial)
1. Baseline exam in all women 35-40 years (30 years in high risk patients)
2. Every 1-2 years between 40-50 years, depending on clinical evaluation, risk factors
3. Annual mammogram after age 50

BREAST DISEASE

BREAST CANCER STAGING

TX	Primary tumor cannot be assessed
T0	No evidence of primary tumor
Tis	Carcinoma in situ; intraductal carcinoma, lobular carcinoma in situ, or Paget's disease of the nipple with no tumor
T1	Tumor 2 cm or less in greatest dimension
T1a	Tumor 0.5 cm but not more than 1 cm in greatest dimension
T1b	Tumor more than 0.5 cm but not more than 1 cm in greatest dimension
T1c	Tumor more than 1 cm but not more than 2 cm in greatest dimension
T2	Tumor more than 2 cm but not more than 5 cm in greatest dimension
T3	Tumor more than 5 cm in greatest dimension
T4	Tumor of any size with direct extension to chest wall or skin
T4a	Extension to chest wall
T4b	Edema (including peau d'orange) or ulceration of the skin of the breast or satellite skin nodules confined to the same breast
T4c	Both T4a and T4b
NX	Regional lymph nodes cannot be assessed (e.g. previously removed)
N0	No regional lymph node metastasis
N1	Metastasis to movable ipsilateral axillary lymph node(s)
N2	Metastasis to ipsilateral axillary lymph node(s), fixed to one another or other structures
N3	Metastasis to ipsilateral mammary lymph node(s)
MX	Presence of distant metastasis cannot be assessed
M0	No evidence of distant metastasis
M1	Distant metastasis, including metastasis to ipsilateral supraclavicular lymph node(s)

Stage	Tumor Size	Lymph node metastasis	Distant metastasis
0	Tis	N0	M0
I	T1	N0	M0
IIa	T0	N1	M0
	T1	N1	M0
	T2	N0	M0
IIb	T2	N1	M0
	T3	N0	M0
IIIa	T0	N2	M0
	T1	N2	M0
	T2	N2	M0
	T3	N1, N2	M0
	T4	Any N	M0
	Any T	N3	M0
IV	Any T	Any N	M1

BREAST CANCER TREATMENT GUIDELINES

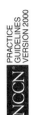

Breast Cancer (noninvasive)

NCCN PRACTICE GUIDELINES VERSION 2000

DIAGNOSIS	WORK-UP	PRIMARY TREATMENT	RISK REDUCTION	SURVEILLANCE/FOLLOW-UP
Lobular carcinoma in situ (LCIS) Stage 0 Tis, N0, M0	• Bilateral mammogram • Pathology review	Observation preferred or In special circumstances: Bilateral mastectomy ± reconstruction may be considered	If treated with observation, counseling regarding use of tamoxifen for risk reduction (category 1, see also NCCN Breast Cancer Risk Reduction Guidelines)	• Interval history and physical exam every 6–12 mo • Mammogram every 12 mo, if observation chosen for primary treatment • If treated with tamoxifen, monitor per NCCN Breast Cancer Risk Reduction Guidelines

Note: All recommendations are category 2A unless otherwise indicated

These guidelines are a work in progress that will be refined as often as new significant data becomes available.

The NCCN guidelines are a statement of consensus of its authors regarding their views of currently accepted approaches to treatment. Any clinician seeking to apply or consult any NCCN guideline is expected to use independent medical judgment in the context of individual clinical circumstances to determine any patient's care or treatment. The National Comprehensive Cancer Network makes no warranties of any kind whatsoever regarding their content, use or application and disclaims any responsibility for their application or use in any way.

Source: National Comprehensive Cancer Network. NCCN Practice Guidelines for Breast Cancer. Reproduced with permission of NCCN. Copyright 2000.

BREAST DISEASE

BREAST CANCER TREATMENT GUIDELINES

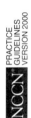

Breast Cancer (noninvasive)

PRACTICE GUIDELINES VERSION 2000

DIAGNOSIS	WORK-UP	PRIMARY TREATMENT	ADJUVANT TREATMENT	SURVEILLANCE/ FOLLOW-UP

Ductal carcinoma in situ (DCIS)[a] Stage 0 Tis, N0, M0

- Bilateral mammogram
- Pathology review

→ **Widespread disease (2 or more quadrants)**

→ **Margins negative[b,c]** → **Small (< 0.5 cm), unicentric, low grade**

Widespread disease (2 or more quadrants):
Total mastectomy without lymph node dissection ± reconstruction[d]
or
Excision + RT
or
Total mastectomy without lymph node dissection ± reconstruction[d,e,f]

Small (< 0.5 cm), unicentric, low grade:
Excision + RT
or
Total mastectomy without lymph node dissection ± reconstruction[d]
or
Excision alone[d,e,f]

Strongly consider tamoxifen for 5 yr:[g]
- Patients treated with breast-conserving therapy (lumpectomy and RT) (category 1)
- Patients treated with excision alone (category 2A)
- Patients treated with mastectomy (category 2B)

- Interval history and physical exam every 6 mo for 5 yr, then annually
- Mammogram every 12 mo
- If treated with tamoxifen, monitor per NCCN Breast Cancer Risk Reduction Guidelines

[a] Clinical trial participation in this situation is especially important.

[b] Re-resection may be necessary to obtain negative margins. Patients not amenable to margin-free excision should have total mastectomy.

[c] Long-term survival with mastectomy vs excision and irradiation appears to be approximately equivalent.

[d] Postexcision specimen radiograph and/or postexcision mammography should document complete tumor excision.

[e] Patients found to have invasive or microinvasive disease at total mastectomy or re-excision should be managed as stage I or II disease, including lymph node dissection.

[f] See treatment contraindications to breast-conserving therapy in the text.

[g] Tamoxifen provides risk reduction in the (ipsilateral breast treated with breast conservation and in the contralateral breast in patients treated with mastectomy or breast conservation. Since a survival advantage has not been demonstrated, individual consideration of risks and benefits is important (see also NCCN Breast Cancer Risk Reduction Guidelines).

Source: National Comprehensive Cancer Network. NCCN Practice Guidelines for Breast Cancer. Reproduced with permission of NCCN. Copyright 2000.

BREAST CANCER TREATMENT GUIDELINES

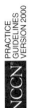

PRACTICE
GUIDELINES
VERSION 2000

Breast Cancer (invasive)

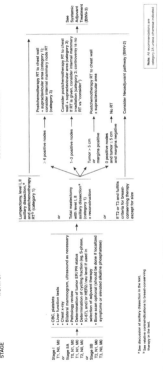

CLINICAL
STAGE

WORK-UP

LOCOREGIONAL TREATMENT

Stage I
T1, N0, M0
or
Stage IIA
T0, N1, M0
T1, N1, M0
T2, N0, M0
or
Stage IIB
T2, N1, M0
T3, N0, M0

• CBC, platelets
• Liver function tests
• Chest x-ray
• Bilateral mammogram, ultrasound as necessary
• Pathology review
• Determination of tumor ER/PR status
• Determination of cycling fraction (eg, S-phase, Ki-67), and/or HER2/neu level if used in selection of adjuvant therapy
• Bone scan optional (should be done if localized symptoms or elevated alkaline phosphatase)

Lumpectomy, level I, II axillary dissection,[a] and postchemotherapy RT[b] (category 1)

or

Total mastectomy with level I, II axillary dissection[a] ± reconstruction (category 1)

or

If T2 or T3 and fulfills criteria for breast-conserving therapy except for size

≥4 positive nodes → Postchemotherapy RT to chest wall + supraclavicular area (category 1); consider internal mammary node RT (category 3)

1–3 positive nodes → Consider postchemotherapy RT to chest wall + supraclavicular area (category 3) If RT is given, consider internal mammary irradiation (category 3; controversy is no RT vs "consider")

Tumor > 5 cm or margins positive → Postchemotherapy RT to chest wall ± supraclavicular area

0 positive nodes and tumor ≤ 5 cm and margins negative → No RT

→ Consider Neoadjuvant pathway (BINV-2)

See Systemic Adjuvant Treatment (BINV-3)

Note: All recommendations are category 2A unless otherwise indicated

[a] See discussion of axillary dissection in the text.
[b] See relative contraindications to breast-conserving therapy in the text.

Source: National Comprehensive Cancer Network, NCCN Practice Guidelines for Breast Cancer. Reproduced with permission of NCCN. Copyright 2000.

BREAST DISEASE

BREAST CANCER TREATMENT GUIDELINES

Neoadjuvant Treatment
Breast Cancer (invasive)

NCCN PRACTICE GUIDELINES VERSION 2000

| CLINICAL STAGE | WORK-UP | PRIMARY TREATMENT | ADJUVANT TREATMENT |

Stage IIIA
T2, N2, M0
or
Stage IIIB
T2, N1, M0
T3, N0, M0

WORK-UP:
- CBC, platelets
- Liver function tests
- Chest x-ray
- Bilateral mammogram, ultrasound as necessary
- Pathology review
- Tumor ER/PR status and HER2/neu level if tumor tissue available
- Bone scan optional (should be done if localized symptoms or elevated alkaline phosphatase) (category 2B)

Anthracycline-based neoadjuvant chemotherapy

No response or Progressive disease → Mastectomy and level I/II axillary dissection ± reconstruction

Partial response, lumpectomy not possible

Core biopsy only

Partial response, lumpectomy possible or Complete response

Desires breast preservation → Lumpectomy with level I/II axillary dissection

Does not desire breast preservation

Individual chemotherapy

Chest wall RT + supraclavicular area; consider internal mammary irradiation (category 2; controversy is "no RT" vs "consider")

Tamoxifen if ER-positive (category 1) If ER-negative, consider tamoxifen for contralateral risk reduction (category 1) → Follow-up

Taxane chemotherapy (category 2B) → Breast and regional lymph node RT

Stage IIIA
T3, N1, M0

WORK-UP:
- CBC, platelets
- Liver function tests
- Chest x-ray
- Pathology review
- Tumor ER/PR status and HER2/neu level if tumor tissue available
- Bilateral mammogram, ultrasound as necessary
- Bone scan (category 2B)
- Abdominal CT/US/MRI (category 2B)

See Stage I and II breast cancer (BINV-1, BINV-3) or Stage III breast cancer (BINV-4)

Source: National Comprehensive Cancer Network, NCCN Practice Guidelines for Breast Cancer. Reproduced with permission of NCCN. Copyright 2000.

176

BREAST CANCER TREATMENT GUIDELINES

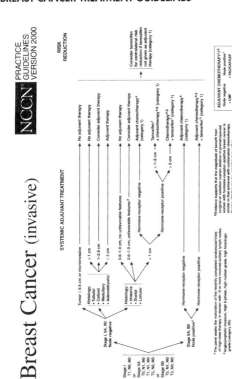

Breast Cancer (invasive)

Source: National Comprehensive Cancer Network. NCCN Practice Guidelines for Breast Cancer. Reproduced with permission of NCCN. Copyright 2000.

BREAST DISEASE

BREAST CANCER TREATMENT GUIDELINES

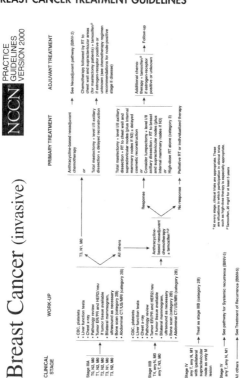

Breast Cancer (invasive)

NCCN PRACTICE GUIDELINES VERSION 2000

CLINICAL STAGE	WORK-UP	PRIMARY TREATMENT	ADJUVANT TREATMENT

Stage IIIA
T0, N2, M0
T1, N2, M0
T2, N2, M0
T3, N1, M0
T3, N2, M0

- CBC, platelets
- Liver function tests
- Chest x-ray
- Pathology review
- Tumor ER/PR and HER2/neu if tumor tissue available
- Bilateral mammogram, ultrasound as necessary
- Bone scan (category 2B)
- Abdominal CT/US/MRI (category 2B)

Stage IIIB
T4, any N, M0
any T, N3, M0

- CBC, platelets
- Liver function tests
- Chest x-ray
- Pathology review
- Tumor ER/PR and HER2/neu if tumor tissue available
- Bilateral mammogram, ultrasound as necessary
- Bone scan (category 2B)
- Abdominal CT/US/MRI (category 2B)

Stage IV
any T, any N, M1 with ipsilateral supraclavicular node as only M lesion → Treat as stage IIIB (category 2B)

Stage IV
any T, any N, M1 → See pathway for Systemic recurrence (BINV-5)

All others → See Treatment of Recurrence (BINV-5)

T3, N1, M0 → Anthracycline-based neoadjuvant chemotherapy
or
Total mastectomy + level I/II axillary dissection ± delayed reconstruction

All others → Anthracycline-based neoadjuvant chemotherapy ± tamoxifen[b] → Response / No response

Response:
Total mastectomy + RT to chest wall and supraclavicular nodes (plus internal mammary nodes if N3) ± delayed cosmetic reconstruction
or
Consider lumpectomy + level I/II axillary dissection + RT to breast and supraclavicular nodes (plus internal mammary nodes if N3)
or
High-dose RT alone (category 3)

No response → Palliative RT or individualized therapy

See Neoadjuvant pathway (BINV-2)

Chemotherapy followed by RT to chest wall and supraclavicular areas (for mastectomy patients) ± tamoxifen[b] if estrogen-receptor positive or unknown (see chemotherapy regimen recommendations for node-positive stage II disease)

Additional chemotherapy + tamoxifen[b] if estrogen-receptor positive or unknown → Follow-up

[a] At every stage, clinical trials are appropriate. These are situations in which participation in clinical trials such as high-dose therapy is especially appropriate.

[b] Tamoxifen, 20 mg/d for at least 5 years

BREAST CANCER TREATMENT GUIDELINES

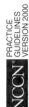

NCCN PRACTICE GUIDELINES VERSION 2000

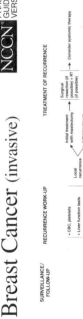

Breast Cancer (invasive)

SURVEILLANCE/FOLLOW-UP

- Interval history and physical exam every 4-6 mo for 5 yr, then every 12 mo
- Mammogram every 12 mo (and 6 mo post-RT if breast-conserving therapy)
- Women on tamoxifen: pelvic exam every 12 mo if uterus present

RECURRENCE WORK-UP

- CBC, platelets
- Liver function tests
- Chest x-ray
- Bone scan
- X-rays of symptomatic bones or bones abnormal on bone scan
- CT or MRI of symptomatic areas
- Biopsy documentation of first recurrence, if possible

TREATMENT OF RECURRENCE

Surgery, radiation, or regional chemotherapy (eg, intrathecal methotrexate) indicated for localized clinical scenarios:
1. Brain metastases
2. Leptomeningeal disease
3. Choroid metastases
4. Pleural effusion
5. Pericardial effusion
6. Biliary obstruction
7. Ureteral obstruction
8. Impending pathologic fracture
9. Pathologic fracture
10. Cord compression
11. Localized painful bone or soft-tissue disease

TREATMENT OF RECURRENCE

Local recurrence → Initial treatment with mastectomy → Surgical resection (if possible) + RT (if possible) → Consider systemic therapy

Local recurrence → Initial treatment with lumpectomy + RT → Mastectomy → Consider systemic therapy

Systemic recurrence → ER/PR positive or bone/soft tissue only or asymptomatic visceral → Prior antiestrogen within 1 yr → Second-line hormonal therapy → Hormone responsive → Additional hormonal therapy

No prior antiestrogen or > 1 yr off antiestrogen → Antiestrogen → Hormone responsive → Additional hormonal therapy

Hormone unresponsive → Chemotherapy

Systemic recurrence → ER/PR negative or symptomatic visceral → Chemotherapy → No response to 2 sequential regimens or ECOG performance status > 3, discontinue chemotherapy (category 2B) → Supportive care

Footnotes:
- Tamoxifen may be given (category 1) in addition to chemotherapy or hormonal therapy if osteolytic lesions, expected survival > 3 months, and creatinine < 2.5 mg/dL.
- Consideration may be given to further hormone therapy in patients failing to respond to first-line hormone therapy and whose disease is indolent, and for those patients achieving a response to chemotherapy and, in whom the decision is made to discontinue chemotherapy.
- See Preferred Chemotherapy Regimens for Recurrent or Metastatic Breast Cancer (Table 2).
- Post-antiestrogen hormonal therapy: selective aromatase inhibitor (anastrozole, letrozole) in postmenopausal women (preferred; category 1); megestrol acetate, fluoxymesterone, ethinyl estradiol or LHRH agonists (premenopausal); surgical or radiotherapeutic oophorectomy (premenopausal)

BREAST DISEASE

BREAST CANCER TREATMENT RISKS

Complication	Risk Factors
Common (affecting >10% of patients)	
Pain or numbness in breast, chest wall or axilla (10-25%)	Greater extent of surgery
Arm swelling or lymphedema (10-25%)	Greater extent of axillary surgery, obesity, weight gain, radiation therapy, infection
Restricted arm motion or weakness (8-10%)	Greater extent of surgery, radiation therapy, recent surgery
Reoperation after breast-implant reconstruction (20-34%)	Radiation therapy
Uncommon (affecting 1-10% of patients)	
Cellulitis	Radiation, seroma
Plexopathy or nerve damage	Higher dose of radiation or larger field
Contralateral breast cancer	Familial or hereditary breast cancer, younger age at diagnosis, higher dose of radiation or larger field
Increased risk of heart disease	Left-sided radiation with older techniques, anthracycline-based chemotherapy
Pneumonitis	Larger radiation field, older age, chemotherapy
Rib fracture	Higher dose of radiation or larger field
Rare (affecting <1% of patients)	
Second cancers other than breast cancer (angiosarcoma, sarcoma, cutaneous cancer, esophageal cancer)	Lymphedema, radiation therapy
Arterial insufficiency	Radiation therapy
Pulmonary fibrosis	Radiation therapy

Broad estimates of incidence reflect different study methods and treatments. Patient surveys typically reveal more frequent symptoms than do chart reviews, although most cases are mild.

Source: Burnstein HJ and Winer EP. Primary care for survivors of breast cancer. *N Engl J Med.* 2000; 343(15):1086-1094. Reproduced with permission of the Massachusetts Medical Society.

BREAST CANCER FOLLOW-UP

Procedure	Frequency
History taking or elicitation of symptoms and examination	Every 3-6 mo for 3 yr, then every 6-12 mo for 2 yr, then annually
Breast self-examination	Monthly
Mammography	Annually
Pelvic examination	Annually
Routine laboratory testing (complete blood count, liver-function tests, automated blood chemical studies, measurement of tumor markers such as CEA, CA 15-3, CA 27.29	Not recommended
Routine radiologic studies (bone scanning, computed tomography, ultrasonography of the liver, chest radiography, pelvic or transvaginal sonography)	Not recommended
Screening for other cancers (e.g., colon, ovarian)	According to recommended guidelines for the general population*

* Women at risk for hereditary breast or ovarian cancer syndromes may merit additional surveillance for ovarian cancer, including pelvic ultrasonography and measurement of serum CA-125 levels, although the benefits of such surveillance are not known.

Treatment of Hot Flashes in Breast Cancer Survivors

Agent	Dose	Type of Drug and Comments
Vitamin E	800 IU daily	Marginal improvement in clinical outcome as compared with placebo.
Megestrol acetate	20 mg twice daily or 500 mg IM every 2 weeks	Progestin; 50-90% of patients report 50% decrease in frequency of hot flashes. Concern about the use of hormonal agent in survivors of breast cancer.
Fluoxetine	20 mg daily	Selective serotonin-reuptake inhibitor; statistically significant reduction in frequency and intensity of hot flashes as compared with placebo.
Venlafaxine	75 mg daily	Selective serotonin-reuptake inhibitor; statistically significant reduction in frequency and intensity of hot flashes as compared with placebo.
Paroxetine	20 mg daily	Selective serotonin-reuptake inhibitor; 67% reduction in number of hot flashes, 75% reduction in intensity score.
Clonidine	Oral or patch, 0.1 mg daily	Antihypertensive; 10-20% reduction in symptoms as compared with placebo; substantial side effects.
Ergotamine and phenobarbital based preparations	Various	No benefit after 8 weeks compared with placebo.
Raloxifene	60 mg daily	Selective estrogen-receptor modulator; no difference in incidence of hot flashes compared with placebo.
Soy phytoestrogens	Daily tablets, each containing 50 mg of soy isoflavones	No improvement in hot flashes as compared with placebo.

Source: Burnstein HJ and Winer EP. Primary care for survivors of breast cancer. *NEJM*. 2000: 343(15):1086-1094. Reproduced with permission of the Massachusetts Medical Society.

CANCER STATISTICS 2000

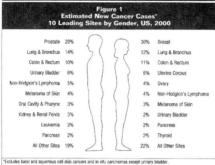

Figure 1
Estimated New Cancer Cases*
10 Leading Sites by Gender, US, 2000

Prostate	29%		30%	Breast
Lung & Bronchus	14%		12%	Lung & Bronchus
Colon & Rectum	10%		11%	Colon & Rectum
Urinary Bladder	6%		6%	Uterine Corpus
Non-Hodgkin's Lymphoma	5%		4%	Ovary
Melanoma of Skin	4%		4%	Non-Hodgkin's Lymphoma
Oral Cavity & Pharynx	3%		3%	Melanoma of Skin
Kidney & Renal Pelvis	3%		2%	Urinary Bladder
Leukemia	3%		2%	Pancreas
Pancreas	2%		2%	Thyroid
All Other Sites	19%		22%	All Other Sites

*Excludes basal and squamous cell skin cancers and in situ carcinomas except urinary bladder.
Percentages may not total 100% due to rounding.

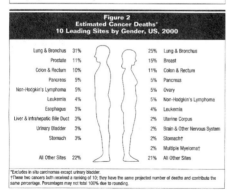

Figure 2
Estimated Cancer Deaths*
10 Leading Sites by Gender, US, 2000

Lung & Bronchus	31%		25%	Lung & Bronchus
Prostate	11%		15%	Breast
Colon & Rectum	10%		11%	Colon & Rectum
Pancreas	5%		5%	Pancreas
Non-Hodgkin's Lymphoma	5%		5%	Ovary
Leukemia	4%		5%	Non-Hodgkin's Lymphoma
Esophagus	3%		4%	Leukemia
Liver & Intrahepatic Bile Duct	3%		2%	Uterine Corpus
Urinary Bladder	3%		2%	Brain & Other Nervous System
Stomach	3%		2%	Stomach†
			2%	Multiple Myeloma†
All Other Sites	22%		21%	All Other Sites

*Excludes in situ carcinomas except urinary bladder.
†These two cancers both received a ranking of 10; they have the same projected number of deaths and contribute the same percentage. Percentages may not total 100% due to rounding.

Source: Greenlee RT, Murray T, Bolden S, Wingo PA. Cancer statistics, 2000. *Ca - A Cancer Journal for Clinicians* 2000;50(1):7-33.
Reproduced with the permission of the American Cancer Society.

GYN-ONCOLOGY

FIGO STAGING AND TREATMENT OF GYNECOLOGIC MALIGNANCIES
Uterine Corpus (surgical staging)

Primary Tumor (T)		
TX	-	Primary tumor cannot be assessed
T0	-	No evidence of primary tumor
Tis	-	Carcinoma *in situ*
T1	I	Tumor confined to corpus uteri
T1a	IA	Tumor limited to endometrium
T1b	IB	Tumor invades up to or less than one-half of myometrium
T1c	IC	Tumor invades to or more than one-half of myometrium
T2	II	Tumor invades cervix but does not extend beyond uterus
T2a	IIA	Endocervical gland involvement only
T2b	IIB	Cervical stroma invasion
T3	III	Local and/or regional spread as specified in T3a, b, and/or N1 and FIGO IIIA, B, and C below
T3a	IIIA	Tumor invades serosa, and/or adnexa, and/or positive peritoneal cytology
T3b	IIIB	Vaginal metastasis
N1	IIIC	Metastasis to pelvis and/or para-aortic lymph nodes
T4	IVA	Tumor invades bladder and/or bowel mucosa
	IVB	Distant metastasis including intraabdominal and/or inguinal lymph nodes

- Notable nuclear atypia raises the grade of a Grade 1 or 2 tumor by 1
- Nuclear grading takes precedence in serous adenocarcinoma, clear-cell adenocarcinoma and squamous cell carcinoma.
- Adenocarcinoma with squamous differentiation are graded according to the nuclear grade of the glandular component

Regional Lymph Nodes (N)	
NX	Regional lymph nodes cannot be assessed
N0	No regional lymph node metastasis
N1	Regional lymph node metastasis

Distant Metastasis (M)	
MX	Distant metastasis cannot be assessed
M0	No distant metastasis
M1	Distant metastasis (including pelvic lymph node metastasis)

GYN-ONCOLOGY

FIGO STAGING AND TREATMENT OF GYNECOLOGIC MALIGNANCIES
Uterine Corpus

Screening

Routine screening of asymptomatic women not recommended.

Diagnosis

Postmenopausal or irregular uterine bleeding. Endometrial and endocervical tissue sample obtained as outpatient or by dilation and curettage under anesthesia.

Pretreatment Work-up

Complete history and physical examination including rectovaginal examination, chest x-ray and CBC, liver and renal function tests as indicated. CT scan, barium enema, CA-125 and bone scan only for patients with suspected metastatic disease.

Staging

Low vertical incision, peritoneal washings or cytologic sampling of ascites, complete abdominal exploration, total abdominal hysterectomy (TAH), bilateral salpingo-oophorectomy (BSO) and pelvic and para-aortic lymph node sampling.

Treatment

TAH + BSO with lymph node sampling is basic treatment for all stages where possible.

Stage I Low risk	Stage I High risk	Stage II	Stage III	Stage IV
• < 1/2 myometrial invasion • Grade 1 or 2	• > 1/2 myometrial invasion •Grade 3 •Lymphatic or vascular invasion	Pelvic radiation followed by TAH/BSO	a. Post primary surgical treatment with no macroscopic residual; post-op pelvic radiation b. Post primary surgical treatment with macroscopic residual; carboplatin/taxol plus irradiation c. Advanced disease unsuitable for surgery; chemotherapy ± radiotherapy	Palliative radiotherapy ± chemotherapy ± hormone therapy
No further treatment after surgical staging	Post-op pelvic irradiation (4,000-5,000 cGy)			

Source: FIGO Committee on Gynecologic Oncology. Gynecologic cancer - staging and guidelines. *Int J Gynaecol Obstet*. 2000; 70(2):209-262.

GYN-ONCOLOGY

FIGO STAGING AND TREATMENT OF GYNECOLOGIC MALIGNANCIES

Cervical Cancer (clinical staging)

(cystoscopy, proctoscopy, IVP, CXR permitted)

Primary Tumor (T)		
TX	-	Primary tumor cannot be assessed
T0	-	No evidence of primary tumor
Tis	-	Carcinoma *in situ* (preinvasive carcinoma)
T1	I	Carcinoma strictly confined to the cervix, corpus extension disregarded
T1a	IA	Invasive carcinoma diagnosed only by microscopy. All macroscopically visible lesions-even with superficial invasion are T1b/IB. Stromal invasion with a maximal depth of 5 mm measured from the base of the epithelium and a horizontal spread of 7 mm or less. Vascular space involvement, venous or lymphatic does not affect classification.
T1a1	IA1	Measured stromal invasion 3 mm or less in depth and 7 mm or less in horizontal spread
T1a2	IA2	Measured stromal invasion more than 3 mm and not more than 5 mm in depth and 7 mm or less in horizontal spread
T1b	IB	Clinically visible lesion confined to the cervix or microscopic lesion greater than T1a2/IA2
T1b1	IB1	Clinically visible lesion 4 cm or less in greatest dimension
T1b2	IB2	Clinically visible lesion more than 4 cm in greatest dimension
T2	II	Cervical carcinoma invades beyond the uterus but not to the pelvic wall or to the lower third of vagina
T2a	IIA	Tumor without parametrial invasion
T2b	IIB	Tumor with parametrial invasion
T3	III	Tumor extends to the pelvic wall and/or involves the lower third of vagina, and/or causes hydronephrosis or non-functioning kidney
T3a	IIIA	Tumor involves lower third of vagina, no extension to pelvic wall
T3b	IIIB	Tumor extends to pelvic wall and/or causes hydronephrosis or non-functioning kidney
T4	IVA	Tumor invades mucosa of bladder or rectum, and/or extends beyond the true pelvis (Bullous edema is not sufficient to classify a tumor as T4)
M1	IVB	Distant metastasis

Regional Lymph Nodes (N)	
NX	Regional lymph nodes cannot be assessed
N0	No regional lymph node metastasis
N1	Regional lymph node metastasis

Distant Metastasis (M)	
MX	Distant metastasis cannot be assessed
M0	No distant metastasis
M1	Distant metastasis (including pelvic lymph node metastasis)

GYN-ONCOLOGY

FIGO STAGING AND TREATMENT OF GYNECOLOGIC MALIGNANCIES
Cervical Cancer

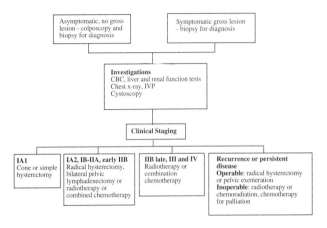

Asymptomatic, no gross lesion - colposcopy and biopsy for diagnosis

Symptomatic gross lesion - biopsy for diagnosis

Investigations
CBC, liver and renal function tests
Chest x-ray, IVP
Cystoscopy

Clinical Staging

IA1
Cone or simple hysterectomy

IA2, IB-IIA, early IIB
Radical hysterectomy, bilateral pelvic lymphadenectomy or radiotherapy or combined chemotherapy

IIB late, III and IV
Radiotherapy or combination chemotherapy

Recurrence or persistent disease
Operable: radical hysterectomy or pelvic exenteration
Inoperable: radiotherapy or chemoradiation, chemotherapy for palliation

Source: FIGO Committee on Gynecologic Oncology. Gynecologic cancer - staging and guidelines. *Int J Gynaecol Obstet* 2000; 70(2):209-262.

GYN-ONCOLOGY

FIGO STAGING AND TREATMENT OF GYNECOLOGIC MALIGNANCIES
Ovarian Cancer

Primary Tumor (T)		
TX	-	Primary tumor cannot be assessed
T0	-	No evidence of primary tumor
T1	I	Tumor limited to ovaries (one or both)
T1a	IA	Growth limited to one ovary, no malignant ascites, no tumor on external surface, capsule intact
T1b	IB	Growth limited to both ovaries, no malignant ascites, no tumor on external surface, capsule intact
T1c	IC	Tumor IA or IB, but positive for surface growth, or malignant ascites, or positive washings, or capsule(s) ruptured at or prior to surgery
T2	II	Tumor involves one or both ovaries with pelvic extension
T2a	IIA	Extension and/or metastases to the uterus and/or tubes. No malignant cells in washings or in ascites.
T2b	IIB	Extension to other pelvic organs. No malignant cells in washings or in ascites.
T2c	IIC	Tumor IIA or IIB, but positive for surface growth, or malignant ascites, or positive washings, or capsule(s) ruptured at or prior to surgery
T3 and/or N1	III	Tumor involving one or both ovaries with microscopic peritoneal implants outside the pelvis and/or positive nodes (retroperitoneal or inguinal). Tumor limited to true pelvis but with histologically proven extension to small bowel and omentum. Superficial liver mets = Stage III
T3a	IIIA	Tumor grossly limited to the true pelvis with negative nodes but microscopic seeding or abdominal peritoneal surface
T3b	IIIB	Tumor with abdominal peritoneal implants but none >2 cm nodes, negative
T3c and/or N1	IIIC	Abdominal implants > 2 cm, and/or positive retroperitoneal or inguinal nodes
M1	IV	Growth involving one or both ovaries with distant mets. Pleural effusions must be tapped for cytology. Parenchymal liver mets = Stage IV

Note: The presence of non-malignant ascites is not classified. The presence of ascites does not affect staging unless malignant cells are present.

Regional Lymph Nodes (N)	
NX	Regional lymph nodes cannot be assessed
N0	No regional lymph node metastasis
N1	Regional lymph node metastasis

Distant Metastasis (M)	
MX	Distant metastasis cannot be assessed
M0	No distant metastasis
M1	Distant metastasis (including pelvic lymph node metastasis)

FIGO STAGING AND TREATMENT OF GYNECOLOGIC MALIGNANCIES
Ovarian Cancer

Screening

Routine screening of asymptomatic women
not recommended.

Diagnosis

Abdominal distention, mass, ascites

Pretreatment Work-up

Complete history and physical examination including pelvic and
rectovaginal examination, chest x-ray and CBC, liver and renal
function tests as indicated. CT scan, ultrasound, barium enema if
indicated. Tumor markers CA-125, CEA, αFP, hCG.

Staging

Staging laparotomy, vertical incision, peritoneal washings or cytologic
sampling of ascites, complete abdominal exploration, total abdominal
hysterectomy (TAH), bilateral salpingo-oophorectomy (BSO) and
pelvic and para-aortic lymph node lymphadenectomy, infracolic
omentectomy, resection of all tumor masses where possible.

Treatment

Low risk	Intermediate Risk	High Risk
• Stages 1a and b • Grade 1 • No residual No further treatment after surgical staging	• Other Stage 1 or II • Grade 2 or 3 • No residual Surgery and chemotherapy carboplatin /paclitaxel for 3-6 cycles	• Any residual • Stage III, IV Surgery and chemotherapy carboplatin /paclitaxel for 6 cycles

Source: FIGO Committee on Gynecologic Oncology. Gynecologic cancer - staging and guidelines. *Int J Gynaecol Obstet.* 2000; 70(2):209-262.

GYN-ONCOLOGY

FIGO STAGING AND TREATMENT OF GYNECOLOGIC MALIGNANCIES
Vulvar (surgical staging)

Primary Tumor (T)	
TX	Primary tumor cannot be assessed
T0	No evidence of primary tumor
Tis	Carcinoma *in situ* (preinvasive carcinoma)
T1	Tumor confined to vulva and/or perineum < 2cm in greatest dimension
T1a	Tumor confined to vulva and/or perineum < 2cm in greatest dimension, and with stromal invasion no greater than 1 mm
T1b	Tumor confined to vulva and/or perineum < 2cm in greatest dimension, and with stromal invasion greater than 1 mm
T2	Tumor confined to vulva and/or perineum > 2cm in greatest dimension
T3	Tumor of any size with adjacent spread to the lower urethra and/or vagina or anus
T4	Tumor invades any of the following: upper urethral mucosa, bladder mucosa, rectal mucosa; or is fixed to the pubic bone

Regional Lymph Nodes (N)	
NX	Regional lymph nodes cannot be assessed
N0	No regional lymph node metastasis
N1	Unilateral regional lymph node metastasis
N2	Bilateral regional lymph node metastasis

Distant Metastasis (M)	
MX	Distant metastasis cannot be assessed
M0	No distant metastasis
M1	Distant metastasis (including pelvic lymph node metastasis)

Stage Grouping

AJCC/UICC/FIGO

0	Tis	N0	M0
IA	T1a	N0	M0
IB	T1b	N0	M0
II	T2	N0	M0
III	T1	N1	M0
	T2	N1	M0
	T3	N0	M0
	T3	N1	M0
IVA	T1	N2	M0
	T2	N2	M0
	T3	N2	M0
	T4	Any N	M0
IVB	Any T	Any N	M1

FIGO STAGING AND TREATMENT OF GYNECOLOGIC MALIGNANCIES

Vulvar (surgical staging)

Screening

Routine screening of asymptomatic
women not recommended.

Diagnosis

Symptomatic, gross lesion seen, biopsy for diagnosis

Pretreatment Work-up

Complete history and physical examination. Chest x-ray, CBC,
liver and renal function tests, ECG as indicated. CT scan,
ultrasound, cystoscopy and barium enema in patients with
suspected metastasis or extension to other organs.

Treatment

VIN	T_{1A}	T_{1B}, T_2	T_{1B}, T_2	T_3, T_4
Wide local excision or CO_2 laser	Microinvasive Wide local excision	(Lateral lesion) Radical local excision with ipsilateral groin dissection or radical hemivulvectomy with *en bloc* ipsilateral inguinal -femoral lymphadenectomy	(Midline lesion) Vulvectomy with *en bloc* bilateral groin dissection or bilateral groin dissection with radical vulvectomy (triple incision technique)	Radical resection pre- or post-irradiation. Rarely exenterative surgery.

Source: FIGO Committee on Gynecologic Oncology. Gynecologic cancer - staging and guidelines. *Int J Gynaecol Obstet.* 2000; 70(2):209-262.

GYN-ONCOLOGY

FIGO STAGING AND TREATMENT OF GYNECOLOGIC MALIGNANCIES
Vagina (clinical staging)

Primary Tumor (T)		
TX	-	Primary tumor cannot be assessed
T0	-	No evidence of primary tumor
Tis	-	Carcinoma *in situ*
T1	I	Tumor confined to vagina
T2	II	Tumor invades paravaginal tissue but not to pelvic wall
T3	III	Tumor extends to pelvic wall
T4*	IVA	Tumor invades bladder and/or bowel mucosa and/or extends beyond the true pelvis (Bullous edema is not sufficient to classify a tumor as T4)
	IVB	Distant metastasis

*Note: If the bladder mucosa is not involved, the tumor is Stage III.

Regional Lymph Nodes (N)	
NX	Regional lymph nodes cannot be assessed
N0	No regional lymph node metastasis
N1	Pelvic or inguinal lymph node metastasis

Distant Metastasis (M)	
MX	Distant metastasis cannot be assessed
M0	No distant metastasis
M1	Distant metastasis (including pelvic lymph node metastasis)

Stage Grouping			
0	Tis	N0	M0
I	T1	N0	M0
II	T2	N0	M0
III	T1	N1	M0
	T2	N1	M0
	T3	N0	M0
	T3	N1	M0
IVA	T4	Any N	M0
IVB	Any T	Any N	M1

Source: FIGO Committee on Gynecologic Oncology. Gynecologic cancer - staging and guidelines. *Int J Gynaecol Obstet.* 2000; 70(2):209-262.

GESTATIONAL TROPHOBLASTIC NEOPLASM

	Partial	Complete	Transitional
Synonym	Incomplete	Classic, true	Blighted ovum
Villi	Crinkled hydropic villi, many normal villi	Pronounced swelling of all villi	Cystic, hydropic, normal
Trophoblast	Mostly syncytial hyperplasia; focal, mild	Cyto- and syncytial hyperplasia is variable	No hyperplasia, may be hypoplasia
Embryo	Usually dies by 9 weeks, may survive to term	Dies very early	Amnion and stunted embryo
Villous capillaries	Many fetal red cells	No fetal red cells	Present
Gestational age	10-22 weeks	8-16 weeks usual	6-14 weeks
hCG titer	75% are < 50,000 mIU/ml	>50,000 mIU/ml usual	Low
Malignant potential	5-10%	15-25%	Slight if any
Karyotype	Triploid (80%)	46XX (95%)	Trisomic, triploidy
Size for dates			
Small	65%	33%	85%
Large	10%	33%	None

Source: Schlaerth JB. Tumors of the placental trophoblast. In: Morrow CP, Curtin JP, Townsend DE, ed. *Synopsis of Gynecologic Oncology*. 4th ed. New York: Churchill Livingstone, 1993. Reproduced with the permission of the publisher.

Signs and symptoms
- first trimester bleeding
- size/date discrepancy
- sudden increase in uterine size
- passage of vesicles
- hyperemesis gravidarum
- early preeclampsia
- thyrotoxicosis
- ß-hCG greater than expected

Good and Poor Prognostic Factors

Good
1. Short duration (last pregnancy < 4 months)
2. Low pretreatment hCG (<40,000 mIU/ml)
3. No brain or liver metastases
4. No significant prior chemotherapy

Poor
1. Long duration (last pregnancy >4 months)
2. High pretreatment hCG (>40,000 mIU/ml)
3. Brain or liver metastases
4. Significant prior chemotherapy
5. Term pregnancy

Outcome

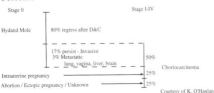

Courtesy of K. O'Hanlan

GYN-ONCOLOGY

POST MOLE SURVEILLANCE

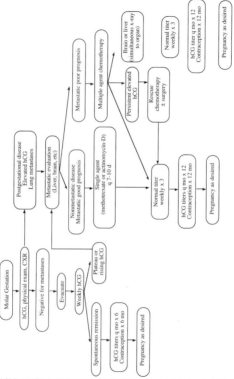

Source: DiSaia PJ, Creasman WT. Gestational trophoblastic neoplasia. In: *Clinical Gynecologic Oncology.* 4th ed. St. Louis: Mosby Year Book, 1993. Reproduced with the permission of the publisher.

GYN-ONCOLOGY

DENNIS SIEGLER'S* TOP TEN WAYS** TO SURVIVE GYN-ONCOLOGY

*   Former Stanford Chief Resident
**   With apologies to David Letterman

10. Do not become angry.
9. DO NOT BECOME ANGRY.
8. **DO NOT BECOME ANGRY.**
7. If angry, do not become frustrated.
6. If angry and frustrated, remember there is always another GOG form to complete.
5. Remember that actual O.R. time = requested O.R. time x 2.
4. Chemotherapy admissions only seem to multiply like rabbits.
3. If all else fails, examine the patient.
2. PM rounds should be completed before AM rounds begin.

And the Number One way to survive Gyn-Onc:

1. Remember, it could be worse; you could be on Internal Medicine

GYN-ONCOLOGY

CHEMOTHERAPY

Drug	Usual Dosage	Acute Side Effects	Toxicity	Precautions	Major Indications
Alkylating Agents					
Cyclophosphamide (Cytoxan)	500-1500 mg/m² IV as a single dose or 60-120 mg/m²/day PO	Nausea/vomiting	Bone marrow depression, alopecia, cystitis	Maintain adequate fluid intake to avoid cystitis	Carcinoma of the cervix, ovary, endometrium, and fallopian tube
Ifosfamide (Ifex)	7-10 g/m² IV over 3-5 days	Nausea/vomiting	Bone marrow depression, alopecia, cystitis	Uroprotector to prevent hemorrhagic cystitis	Carcinoma and sarcoma of the ovary, cervix, and endometrium. Germ cell tumors.
Cycle-specific Antimetabolites					
5-Fluorouracil (5-FU)	12 mg/kg/day IV for 4 days, then alternate days at 6 mg/kg for 4 days or until toxicity; repeat course monthly or give weekly IV dose of 12-15 mg/kg; maximal dose 1 g for either regimen; often used in combination regimens at a dose of 500 mg/m² IV	Occasional nausea/vomiting	Bone marrow depression, diarrhea, stomatitis, alopecia	Decrease dose in patients with diminished liver, renal, or bone marrow function or after adrenalectomy	Carcinoma of the ovary and endometrium
Methotrexate (MTX, Amethopterin)	Choriocarcinoma: 10-30 mg/m² q day IV for 5 days. Ovarian or cervical carcinoma: 200-2000 mg/m² IV with leukovorin rescue	None	Bone marrow depression, megaloblastic anemia, diarrhea, stomatitis, vomiting, alopecia less common; occasional hepatic fibrosis, vasculitis, pulmonary fibrosis	Adequate renal function must be present and urine output must be maintained	Choriocarcinoma, carcinoma of the cervix and ovary
Cytarabine (Ara-C, Cytosar-U)	200 mg/m² daily for 5 days by continuous infusion	Nausea/vomiting	Bone marrow depression, megaloblastosis, leukopenia, thrombocytopenia	None	Carcinoma of the ovary (intraperitoneal use)
Gemcitabine (Gemzar) (2,2-difluorodeoxycystabidine)	800-1000 mg/m² IV weekly every 3 weeks	Mild nausea, vomiting, malaise (usually mild), transient febrile episodes, maculopapular rash)	Bone marrow suppression	None	Carcinoma of the breast and ovary

Source: DiSaia PJ, Creasman WT. Basic principles of chemotherapy. In: *Clinical Gynecologic Oncology*. 5th ed. St. Louis: Mosby Year Book; 1997. Reproduced with the permission of the publisher.

CHEMOTHERAPY (CONT.)

Drug	Usual Dosage	Acute Side Effects	Toxicity	Precautions	Major Indications
Antibiotics					
Dactinomycin (Cosmegen)	15 mcg/kg/day IV or 0.5 mg/day for 5 days	Pain on local infiltration with skin necrosis; nausea and vomiting in many patients after 2 hours; occasional cramps and diarrhea	Bone marrow depression, stomatitis, diarrhea, erythema, hyperpigmentation with occasional desquamation in areas of previous radiation	Administer through running IV infusion; use with care in liver disease and in presence of inadequate marrow function; prophylactic antiemetics are helpful	Embryonal rhabdomyosarcoma, choriocarcinoma, ovarian germ cell tumors
Mitomycin-C (Mutamycin)	0.05 mg/kg/day IV for 6 days, then alternate days until 50 mg total dose	Nausea, vomiting, local inflammation and ulceration if extravasated	Neutropenia, thrombocytopenia, oral ulceration, nausea, vomiting and diarrhea	Administer through running IV infusion or inject with great care to prevent extravasation	Carcinoma of the cervix
Bleomycin (Blenoxane)	10-20 mg/m² IV or IM 1-2x weekly	Nausea/vomiting, fever, chills, local pain and phlebitis less frequent	Skin hyperpigmentation, thickening, nail changes, ulceration, rash, peeling, alopecia Pulmonary: pneumonitis with dyspnea, rales, infiltrate can progress to fibrosis; more common in patients over 70 and with more than 400 mg total dose, but unpredictable	Watch for hypersensitivity in lymphoma in first 1-2 doses; use with extreme caution in presence of renal or pulmonary disease; start in hospital under observation; do not exceed 400 mg total dose	Squamous cell carcinoma of the cervix, vulva and skin; choriocarcinoma
Doxorubicin (Adriamycin)	60-100 mg/m² IV every 3 weeks	Nausea/vomiting, fever, local phlebitis, necrosis if extravasated, red urine (not blood)	Bone marrow depression, alopecia, cardiac toxicity related to cumulative dose, stomatitis, atrophy of the myocardium can occur, especially if a total dose of 450-500 mg/m² is exceeded	Administer through running IV infusion; avoid giving to patients with significant heart disease; follow for ECG abnormalities and signs of heart failure	Adenocarcinoma of the endometrium, fallopian tube, ovary and vagina; uterine sarcoma

Source: DiSaia PJ, Creasman WT. Basic principles of chemotherapy. In: *Clinical Gynecologic Oncology*. 5th ed. St. Louis: Mosby Year Book, 1997. Reproduced with the permission of the publisher.

GYN-ONCOLOGY

CHEMOTHERAPY (CONT.)

Drug	Usual Dosage	Acute Side Effects	Toxicity	Precautions	Major Indications
Plant Alkaloids					
Vinblastine (Velban)	0.10-0.15 mg/kg/week IV	Severe, prolonged inflammation if extravasated, occasional nausea, vomiting, headache, and paresthesias	Bone marrow depression, particularly neutropenia, alopecia, muscle weakness, occasional mild peripheral neuropathy, mental depression 2-3 days after treatment, rarely stomatitis	Administer through running IV infusion to prevent extravasation; decrease dose in liver disease	Choriocarcinoma
Vincristine (Oncovin)	0.4-1.4 mg/m² /week IV	Local inflammation if extravasated	Paresthesias, weakness, loss of reflexes, constipation; abdominal, chest, and jaw pain, hoarseness, foot drop; mental depression, marrow toxicity generally mild, anemia and reticulocytopenia most prominent, alopecia	Administer through running IV infusion or inject with great care to prevent extravasation; decrease dose in liver disease; patients with underlying neurologic problems may be more susceptible to neurotoxicity; alopecia may be prevented by the use of a scalp tourniquet for 5 minutes during and after administration	Uterine sarcoma, germ cell tumor of the ovary
Etoposide (VP-16, VePesid)	100 mg/m² IV days 1,3,5 q 4 weeks	Nausea and vomiting	Leukopenia, thrombocytopenia, alopecia, headache, fever, occasional hypotension	Reduce dose by 25-50% for hematologic toxicity	Trophoblast disease; germ cell tumors
Paclitaxel (Taxol)	170-250 mg/m² IV every 3-4 weeks	Allergic reaction, nausea, vomiting	Bone marrow depression, severe allergic-like reactions with facial erythema, dyspnea, tachycardia, and hypotension cardiotoxicity with bradycardia, alopecia, stomatitis, fatigue	Cardiac monitoring may be necessary	Ovarian carcinoma
Vinorelbine tartrate (Navelbine)	30 mg/m2 weekly IV	Mild nausea, 10% alopecia	Bone marrow depression, mild to moderate peripheral neuropathy	Local irritant, dose modification with hepatic dysfunction	Ovarian carcinoma

Source: DiSaia PJ, Creasman WT. Basic principles of chemotherapy. In: *Clinical Gynecologic Oncology*. 5th ed. St. Louis: Mosby Year Book; 1997. Reproduced with the permission of the publisher.

CHEMOTHERAPY (CONT.)

Drug	Usual Dosage	Acute Side Effects	Toxicity	Precautions	Major Indications
Miscellaneous					
Hydroxyurea (Hydrea)	80 mg/kg PO q 3 day 20-30 mg/kg PO daily	Anorexia and vomiting	Bone marrow depression, megaloblastic anemia; stomatitis, diarrhea, and alopecia less common	Decrease dose in patients with marrow and renal dysfunction	Carcinoma of the cervix (with radiotherapy)
Cisplatin (CDDP, Platinol)	50-100 mg/m² IV q 3 weeks	Nausea and vomiting often severe	Renal damage; moderate myelosuppression; severe renal damage can be minimized by not exceeding a total dose of 500 mg/m² in any treatment course	Infuse at a rate not to exceed 1 mg/min and only after 10-12 hours of hydration; avoid nephrotoxic antibiotics; watch renal function and discontinue if BUN exceeds 30 or creatinine exceeds 2	Carcinoma of the ovary, endometrium, or cervix
Carboplatin (Paraplatin)	250-400 mg/m² IV bolus or by 24-hr continuous infusion every 2-4 weeks	Mild nausea and vomiting	Bone marrow suppression, especially thrombocytopenia	Decreased dose in patients who have had previous chemotherapy	Carcinoma of the ovary, endometrium, or cervix
Hexamethylmelamine (Hexalen)	4-12 mg/kg/day PO in divided doses for 14-21 days, repeated every 6 weeks	Nausea and vomiting	Bone marrow depression, neurotoxicity, both central and peripheral	None	Ovarian carcinoma
Dacarbazine (DTIC)	80-160 mg/m²/day x 10 d	Nausea and vomiting	Bone marrow depression	Patients may develop severe nausea and vomiting	Uterine sarcoma
Hycamptamine (Topotecan)	1.5 mg/m² daily for 5 days	Maculopapular pruritic exanthema	Bone marrow depression	Watch for neutropenia fever	Ovarian carcinoma
Progestational Agents					
Medroxyprogesterone acetate (Provera)	400-800 mg/week IM or PO	None	Occasional liver function abnormalities; occasional alopecia and hypersensitivity reactions	Use with care in presence of liver dysfunction	Carcinoma of the endometrium
Hydroxyprogesterone caproate	1000 mg IM 2x/week				
Megestrol acetate (Megace)	20-80 mg PO bid				

Source: DiSaia PJ, Creasman WT. Basic principles of chemotherapy. In: *Clinical Gynecologic Oncology*. 5th ed. St. Louis: Mosby Year Book; 1997. Reproduced with the permission of the publisher.

GYN-ONCOLOGY

BOWEL PREP (USUALLY FOR OVARIAN CANCER CASES)
Teng Recipe
1. Golytely with 1-2 cups juice per liter. 4 liters PO (8 ounces q 10 min)
2. Cefotetan 2 g IV q 12 hr, give in PM and 1 hr prior to operation
3. Soap Suds Enema night before and in AM until clear

O'Hanlan Recipe
Ovarian cancer or advanced laparoscopy
1. Golytely (add powder to 3 liters of water and 500-1000 cc apple juice)
2. Cefotetan 2 g IV and Flagyl 500 mg IV one hour prior to surgery
3. Clear liquids after 3 PM, NPO after midnight on day before surgery
   (IV after midnight for inpatients)

Endometrial/cervical cancer.
1. Fleet's enema at bedtime and in the morning

DAILY ONCOLOGY PROGRESS NOTE
Should always include the following information
- vital signs
- weight (previous weight)
- I/O = PO + IV/Foley + NG + Drains
- meds: list all meds **including** IVF with rate
- labs: if new, list all; if previously recorded, list as normal CBC, GSP, etc. and
  summarize abnormal values (e.g. SGOT 800 on 3/14, now 250)
- exam: be brief but meticulous
- impression/plan: problem oriented by system
  - fluids, electrolytes, nutrition (FEN)
  - cardiovascular
  - hematologic
  - respiratory
  - renal
  - gastrointestinal
  - infection
  - neurologic

PRE-OPERATIVE CHECKLIST
1. Check with operating room (O.R.) regarding schedule
2. Check all labs (call Attending if any questionable values)
3. Obtain EKG, CXR (if indicated)
4. Begin heparin 5000 units SQ BID prior to surgery
5. Order S.C.D./T.E.D. hose
6. Cefotetan 2 g IV on call to O.R.
7. Obtain consent personally and have patient sign any other forms
8. Discuss autologous or donor directed blood prior to day of surgery
9. Write Pre-op Note with labs, planned procedure, consent

IV FLUID COMPOSITION

	Na$^+$	Cl$^-$	K$^+$	HCO$_3^-$	Ca^{+2}	Glucose	Amino acids	Mg^{+2}	PO$_4^{-3}$	Acetate	Osm
Extracellular fluid	140	102	4.0	28	5.0						290
Normal saline	154	154									308
1/2 Normal saline	77	77									154
1/4 Normal saline	34	34									78
Lactated Ringers	130	109	4.0	28	3.0						272
D5W						50 g					252
D10W						100 g					505
Peripheral parenteral nutrition	47	40	13			100 g	35 g	3.0	3.5	52	500
Total parenteral nutrition	25	30	44			250 g	50 g	5.0	15	99	190
D50						500 g					

BODY FLUID COMPOSITION

	Na$^+$	Cl$^-$	K$^+$	HCO$_3^-$	Daily Production (mL)
Gastric juices	60-100	100	10	0	1500-2000
Duodenum	130	90	5	0-10	300-2000
Bile	145	100	5	15-35	100-800
Pancreatic juices	140	75	5	70-115	100-800
Ileum	140	100	5	15-30	2000-3000

GYN-ONCOLOGY

NUTRITIONAL REQUIREMENTS
Caloric Requirements
• Basal energy expenditure (BEE): energy expended under complete rest (in kcal):

   Males = 66 + [13.8 x weight (kg)] + [5 x height (cm)] - [6.8 X age (years)]

   Females = 65 + [13.8 x weight (kg)] + [5 x height (cm)] - [6.8 X age (years)]

• Injury factor (IF): used to adjust BEE for effects of disease process

Mild starvation/postoperative	BEE + 10%
Multiple trauma and ventilator or sepsis	BEE + 40%
Cancer	BEE + 20%
Long-bone fracture	BEE + 30%
Fever	BEE + 13%

ª Activity factor (AF): used to adjust BEE

Bed rest	1.2
Out of bed	1.3

• Total daily expenditure (TDE): total energy expended per day

   TDE = BEE x IF x AF (kcal/day)

Comments
• Caloric requirements are met from carbohydrates and fat (not protein)
• Dextrose: 3.4 kcal/g
• Lipids: 9 kcal/g; need to provide at least 4% calories as linoleic acid
• Amino acid: 4 kcal/g (although usually not included in caloric calculations)

Protein Requirements

Minimal	0.5 g/kg/day
RDA	0.8 g/kg/day
Trauma, sepsis	1.5-3.0 g/kg/day
Acute renal failure	0.5-0.8 g/kg/day
Hemodialysis	1.0-1.5 g/kg/day
Peritoneal dialysis	1.5 g/kg/day

Fluid Requirements
• 1.0 ml/calorie/day
• 30 ml/kg/day

Source: Nutrition Services, Stanford University Hospital. *Adult TPN Handbook.* Stanford, CA: Stanford University Hospital, 1996.

TOTAL PARENTERAL NUTRITION
Indications
Definite Benefit
- Inability to use the GI tract
        Massive bowel resection
        Severe diarrhea
        Diseases of the small intestine
        Intractable vomiting
        Radiation enteritis
- Severely catabolic when the GI tract is unusable for 5-7 days
- Severe malnutrition with a nonfunctional GI tract
- Undergoing high-dose chemotherapy, radiation thereapy, bone marrow transplantation
- Moderate to severe acute pancreatitis

Probable Benefit
- major surgery: NPO expected for 7-10 days
- Moderate stress: enteral feeding not tolerated for 7-10 days
- High output enterocutaneous fistula (e.g.,>500 mL/day)
- Inflammatory bowel disease with nonfunctional GI tract
- Small-bowel obstruction
- Hyperemesis gravidarum

Peripheral Parenteral Nutrition (PPN) Nutrition
- Expected duration of parenteral therapy is < 7 days
- Temporary loss of GI function (e.g., acute ileus)
- Maximum concentration of PPN should not exceed dextrose 10% + amino acids 4.25% and concurrent lipid infusion to decrease vein irritation

Complications of Total Parenteral Nutrition
- Hyperglycemia
- Hypoglycemia
- Electrolyte disorders (PO_4, K)
- Mineral deficiency (Mg, Zn)
- Vitamin deficiency
- Trace element deficiency
- Essential fatty acid deficiency
- Hyperlipidemia
- Metabolic acidosis
- Heart failure
- Anemia
- Demineralization of bone
- Steatosis
- Cholestasis
- Sepsis (especially fungemia)
- Respiratory failure

GYN-ONCOLOGY

STEROIDS

Generic Name	Trade Name	Relative Potency			Starting Doses (mg)	
		Glucocorticoid and anti-inflammatory	Mineralo-corticoid	Equivalent doses (mg)	Moderate illness	Severe illness
Short-acting						
Hydrocortisone (cortisol)	Cortef Solu-Cortef	1	1	20	80-160	
Cortisone		0.8	0.8	25	100-200	
Prednisone	Deltasone Meticorten	4	0.8	5	20-40	60-100
Prednisolone	Delta-Cortef Meticortelone	4	0.8	5	20-40	60-100
Methylprednisolone	Medrol Solu-Medrol	5	0.5	4	16-32	48-80
Intermediate-acting						
Triamcinolone	Aristocort Kenacort	5	0	4	16-32	48-80
Paramethasone	Haldrone	10	0	2	8-16	24-40
Long-acting						
Dexamethasone	Decadron	25	0	0.75	3-6	9-15
Betamethasone	Celestone	25	0	0.6	2.4-4.8	7.2-12

Source: Klearman M, Pereira M. Arthritis and rheumatologic diseases. In: Dunagan WC, Ridner ML, ed. *Manual of Medical Therapeutics*. 27th ed. Boston: Little, Brown, 1992. Reproduced with the permission of the publisher.

HANDY FORMULAS

$$\text{Creatinine Clearance} = \frac{(0.85)\,(\text{wt in kg})\,(140 - \text{age})}{72 \times \text{serum creatinine}}$$

$$FE_{Na} = \frac{U_{Na} \times S_{Cr}}{S_{Na} \times U_{Cr}} \times 100$$

1 Kcal / cc of D25 HAL; 1 Kcal / cc of 10% Lipids

Real [Na] = measured [Na] + 0.16 (serum glucose)

$$\text{Iron Dextran} = \frac{100 \text{ mg } Fe^{2+}}{2 \text{ cc}} \qquad \text{Fe deficit} = 1000 + (15 - \text{Hgb})\,(\text{wt in kg})$$

$$\text{Osmolality} = 2\,[\text{Na}] + [\text{K}] + \frac{BUN}{2.8} + \frac{\text{Glucose}}{18} \qquad \text{Normal (280-295)}$$

A-a Gradient = P_{AO_2} - P_{aO_2} = <15 mm Hg in healthy, young person

$$P_{AO_2} = FiO_2 \times (PB - PH_2O) - PaCO_2 / R$$

FiO_2 = Fractional [ ] of inspired O_2
PB = Barometric pressure (760 mm Hg @ sea level)
PH_2O = water vapor pressure (47 mm Hg when fully sat.)
R   = resp. quotient (rate of CO_2 prod. to O_2 consumption, usually assumed to be 0.8)

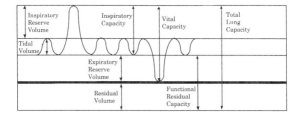

GYN-ONCOLOGY

INVASIVE CARDIAC MONITORING

Fast Facts
• Swan-Ganz catheter allows accurate measurement of hemodynamic parameters in acutely ill patient
• introduced into clinical practice in 1970

Indications
Sepsis with refractory hypotension or oliguria
Unexplained or refractory pulmonary edema, heart failure or oliguria
Severe PIH with pulmonary edema or oliguria
Intraoperative or intrapartum cardiovascular decompensation
Massive blood loss and volume loss or replacement
Adult respiratory distress syndrome (ARDS)
Shock of undefined etiology
Some chronic conditions, particularly associated with labor or surgery
    • NYHA Class III or IV cardiac disease (structural or physiologic)
    • Peripartum or perioperative coronary artery disease (ischemia, infarction)

Triple lumen

Distal port (red): located in pulmonary artery. Attached to pressure transducer to provide continuous PAP tracings and allow PCWP determination. Can also withdraw mixed venous blood from pulmonary artery.

Proximal port (blue): located in superior vena cava. Can be used in infuse fluids and also used in cardiac output measurements.

Thermistor: a temperature sensor used in determination of cardiac output.

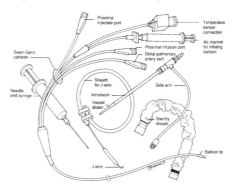

Source: Mabie WC. Critical care obstetrics. In: Gabbe SG, Niebyl JR, Simpson JL, ed. *Obstetrics : normal and problem pregnancies.* 2nd ed. New York: Churchill Livingstone, 1991. Reproduced with the permission of the publisher.

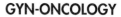

INVASIVE CARDIAC MONITORING

Wedge pressure
A measurement of left ventricular preload. The pulmonary artery wedge pressure is obtained with a balloon-tipped catheter advanced into a branch of pulmonary artery until the vessel is occluded, forming a free communication through the pulmonary capillaries and veins to the left atrium. A true wedge position is in the lung zone where both pulmonary artery and pulmonary venous pressures exceed alveolar pressure.

Preload
Initial stretch of the myocardial fiber at end diastole. Clinically the right and left ventricular end-diastolic pressures are assessed by the central venous pressure and wedge pressure respectively.

Afterload
Wall tension of the ventricle during ejection. Best reflected by systolic blood pressure.

Contractility
The force of myocardial contractility when preload and after load are held constant.

Derivation of hemodynamic parameters

Mean arterial pressure	MAP	mm Hg	$\frac{\text{systolic pressure} + 2 \ (\text{diastolic pressure})}{3}$
Stroke volume	SV	ml/beat	CO / HR
Stroke index	SI	ml/beat/m2	SV / BSA
Cardiac index	CI	L/min/m2	CO / BSA
Pulmonary vascular resistance	PVR	dynes x s x cm-5	$\frac{\text{MPAP - PCWP}}{\text{CO}} \times 80$
Systemic vascular resistance	SVR	dynes x s x cm-5	$\frac{\text{MAP - CVP}}{\text{CO}} \times 80$

Normal hemodynamic values

Parameter	Nonpregnant	Trimester of Pregnancy		
		1st	2nd	3rd
Heart beat (beats/min)	60-100	81	84	84
Central venous pressure (mm Hg)	5-10			
Mean pulmonary artery wedge pressure (mm Hg)	15-20			
Pulmonary capillary wedge pressure (mm Hg)	6-12			
Mean arterial pressure (mm Hg)	90-110	82	84	86
Cardiac output (L/min)	4.3-6.0	6.2	6.3	6.4
Stroke volume (mL/beat)	57-71	76	75	76
Systemic vascular resistance (dynes x sec x cm⁻³)	900-1400	1087	1093	1119
Pulmonary vascular resistance (dynes x sec x cm⁻⁵)	<250			

Adapted with permission from Clark SL, Cotton DB, Lee W, et al Central hemodynamic assessment of normal term pregnancy. *Am J Obstet Gynecol.* 1989;161(6 Pt 1):1439-42 and Rosenthal MH. Intrapartum intensive care management of the cardiac patient. *Clin Obstet Gynecol.* 1981;24(3):789-807.

GYN-ONCOLOGY

INVASIVE HEMODYNAMIC MONITORING

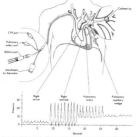

Source: Gibson RS, Kistner JR. Swan-Ganz catheter insertion. In: Suratt PM, Gibson RS, ed. *Manual of Medical Procedures*. St. Louis: Mosby, 1982. Reproduced with the permission of the publisher.

HEMODYNAMIC THERAPY

	Decreased	Increased
Preload		
	Crystalloid Colloid Blood	**Diuretics** furosemide ethacrynic acid mannitol
		Venodilators furosemide nitroglycerin morphine
Afterload		
	Volume Inotropic support Vasopressors norepinephrine phenylephrine metaraminol	**Arterial dilators** hydralazine diazoxide
		Venous dilators nitroglycerin
		Mixed arteriovenous dilators nitroprusside trimethaphan
Contractility		
	Dopamine Dobutamine Epinephrine Calcium Digitalis	

Source: Gomella LG, Braen GR, Olding MJ. Critical care. In: *Clinician's Pocket Reference : the scut monkey's handbook*. 7th ed. Norwalk, Conn.: Appleton & Lange, 1993. Reproduced with the permission of the publisher.

AFTER MIDNIGHT ABC'S FOR GYN-ONC
Key Points
• Good sign out
• Get to know the patient before ordering tests
• Make the diagnosis quickly... minutes can make a difference
• Avoid wishful thinking

  "If you wait, then the patient will get better... they never do"
  Teng 1991

I. THROMBOEMBOLIC PHENOMENA
Signs and Symptoms
• 90% tachypnea
• 45% tachycardia
• 30% hemoptysis
• 20% cyanosis

Physical Exam
• evaluate for pulmonary compromise
• lower extremities for evidence of deep vein thrombosis (DVT)

Evaluation

• ABG PO_2 often < 80, but don't get fooled
• EKG changes often unreliable, RBB, right axis shift (S1Q3T3) in extensive embolization
• CXR atelectasis, raised hemidiaphragm, pulmonary effusions
• V/Q Scan will give low, intermediate, or high probability of PE
  If intermediate, then consider angiogram.

Treatment
• O_2 titrate to keep O_2 sat > 92
• heparin 10,000 units bolus, 1000 units/hr to keep PTT 1.5-2x normal
• coumadin started after 4-7 days on heparin
    • give 10 mg, 10 mg, 10 mg, 5 mg
    • follow PT (keep 1.5-2.0x normal)

DVT/PE Prophylaxis
• heparin 5000 units SQ q 12 hr
• q 8 hr if obese
• S.C.D./T.E.D. hose post operatively
• Do not D/C the above prophylaxis until ambulating well

GYN-ONCOLOGY

II. SEPSIS SYNDROME

Definition:
• Clinical syndrome of systemic toxicity (sepsis) related to infection which often leads to CV collapse

Fast Facts:
• 70-80% are the result of gram-negative bacteria
• 70,000-300,000 cases annually
• 30-50% of episodes associated with septic shock
• mortality rate approaches 30%

Diagnosis:
Each of the following four:
• clinical evidence to support a presumptive diagnosis of gram-negative infection, and evidence of deleterious systemic effects.
• core temperature T>38.3°C (101°F) or unexplained hypothermia <35.6° C
• tachycardia (>90 bpm) in absence of ß-blockade and tachypnea (RR>20 or requiring mechanical ventilation)
• hypotension (SBP 90 mm Hg or drop in SBP 40 mm Hg) in presence of adequate volume status and no antihypertensive agents.

Or

Evidence of systemic toxicity or poor end-organ perfusion defined by at least two of the following:
• unexplained metabolic acidosis (pH < 7.3, a base deficit of > 5, or increased plasma lactate)
• arterial hypoxia (PO_2 75 mm Hg or PO $_2$/FiO_2 ratio < 250) in patient without overt pulmonary disease.
• acute renal failure (UO < 30 cc/hr) for 1 hour despite acute volume loading and evidence of adequate intravascular volume.
• recent (within 24 hr) unexplained coagulation abnormalities (increased PT/PTT) or unexplained platelet depression (<100,000 or decrease of 50% from baseline)
• mental status changes
• elevated cardiac index (> 4/L/min/m²) with low SVR (<800 dyne-sec/cm⁵)

Management
1) History and physical exam
2) Volume replacement
3) Blood/urine/sputum cultures
4) O_2, labs, x-rays (CXR, KUB, etc.)
5) Broad spectrum antibiotics
6) Consider transfer to ICU for pressor support

GYN-ONCOLOGY

III. EXTRAVASATION INJURY

Class/Specific Agent	Local Antidote	Specific Procedure
Alkylating Agents		
Cisplatin, Mechlorethamine	1/3 or 1/6 M sodium thiosulfate	Mix 4-8 ml 10% sodium thiosulfate U.S.P. with 6 ml of sterile water for injection, U.S.P. for a 1/3 or 1/6 M solution. Inject 2 ml into site for each mg of mechlorethamine or 100 mg of cisplatin extravasated.
Mitomycin-C	Dimethylsulfoxide (DMSO) 50-99% (w/v)	Apply 1.5 ml to the site every 6 hours for 14 days. Allow to air-dry, do not cover
DNA intercalators		
Doxorubicin, Daunorubicin, Amsacrine	Cold compresses	Apply immediately for 30-60 minutes, then alternate on/off every 15 minutes for 1 day.
	Dimethylsulfoxide (DMSO) 50-99% (w/v)	Apply 1.5 ml to the site every 6 hours for 14 days. Allow to air-dry, do not cover.
Vinca alkaloids		
Vinblastine, Vincristine	Warm compresses Hyaluronidase	Apply immediately for 30-60 minutes, then alternate on/off every 15 minutes for 1 day. Inject 150 U hyaluronidase (Wydase, others) into site.
Epipodophyllotoxins		
Etoposide, Teniposide	Warm compresses Hyaluronidase	Apply immediately for 30-60 minutes, then alternate on/off every 15 minutes for 1 day. Inject 150 U hyaluronidase (Wydase, others) into site.

Source: Dorr RT. Pharmacologic management of vesicant chemotherapy extravasations. In: Dorr RT, Von Hoff DD, ed. *Cancer Chemotherapy Handbook*. 2nd ed. Norwalk, Conn.: Appleton & Lange, 1994. Reproduced with the permission of the publisher.

IV. ABDOMINAL DEHISCENCE

Predisposing Factors:
- inadequate closure
- previous radiation
- infection (cellulitis must be examined)
- poor nutrition (albumin < 3.0)
- obesity
- immunocompromised (steroid use)
- diabetes
- smoker

Signs and Symptoms:
- sudden wound discomfort or none at all
- sensation of disruption by patient
- appearance of copious, persistent serosanguinous wound drainage
- prolonged paralytic ileus
  THESE SIGNS REPRESENT DEHISCENCE UNTIL PROVEN OTHERWISE

Management:
- semi-Fowler's position
- cover bowels/wound with sterile, wet gauze pads
- place NG tube to decompress bowel
- initiate broad spectrum antibiotic coverage
- plan for surgical closure if operative candidate

GYN-ONCOLOGY

V. HEMORRHAGE

"Hypovolemia is a problem."
Teng, 1991

Unsatisfactory Hemostasis
Signs and Symptoms
• can be revealed or concealed
• tachycardia, ectopy, chest pain
• cold extremities
• confusion secondary to hypoxia
• abdominal distention
• hemoperitoneum
EARLY RECOGNITION IS CRUCIAL

Management
• medical stabilization
• surgical re-exploration

Coagulopathy
Signs and Symptoms
• unexplained bleeding from wound, IV sites, etc.
• red top tube fails to clot
• microangiopathic changes revealed on DIC panel

Management
• correction of underlying cause
• sepsis, fetal demise, tissue necrosis, replacement of blood products

GI Bleeding
Etiology
• ulcers
• XRT (proctitis)
• catheter erosion
• varices
• Mallory-Weiss tears

Management
• identify source
• H2 blockers, gastric lavage
• angiography with embolization

Blood Products

Component	Contents	Volume	Indication
Packed red blood cells	Red cells with most plasma removed	1 unit = 250-300 cc 1 unit raises Hct by 3%	Acute or chronic blood loss
Platelets	Platelets only	One pack = 50 cc One pack raises platelets by 6K; six-pack is from 6 donors' blood	Platelets < 20 K in non-bleeding patient Platelets < 50 K in bleeding patient
Fresh frozen plasma (FFP)	Fibrinogen, Factors II, VII, IX, X, XI, XII, XIII, and heat labile V and VII	1 unit = 150 - 250 cc 11 g albumin 500 mg fibrinogen 0.7-1.0 units clotting factors	DIC, transfusion > 10 units Liver disease, IgG deficiency 1 unit raises fibrinogen by 10 mg/dL
Cryoprecipitated antihemophilic factor (Cryo)	Factors VIII, XIII, von Willebrand's, fibrinogen	1 unit = 10 cc 250 mg fibrinogen 80 units factor VIII	Hemophilia A, von Willebrand's disease, fibrinogen deficiency

VI. ACID/BASE DISTURBANCES

Interpretation of ABG's:

Rule I: A change in PCO_2 down or up of 10 mm Hg is associated with an increase or decrease of pH of 0.08 units.

Rule II: A pH change of 0.15 is equivalent to a base change of 10 mEq/L

Rule III: The dose of bicarbonate (in mEq) required to fully correct a metabolic acidosis is

$$\frac{\text{Base deficit (mEq/L) x patient weight (kg)}}{4}$$

Rule IV: If the alveolar ventilation increases, PCO_2 will decrease, if alveolar ventilation decreases, PCO_2 will increase.

Source: Gomella LG, Braen GR, Olding MJ. Blood gases and acid base disorders. In: *Clinician's Pocket Reference: the Scut Monkey's Handbook.* 7th ed. Norwalk, Conn.: Appleton & Lange, 1993. Reproduced with the permission of the publisher.

Differential Diagnosis

	pH	HCO_3	PCO_2
Metabolic acidosis	↓	↓↓	
Metabolic alkalosis	↑	↑↑	↑
Respiratory acidosis	↓	↑	↑↑
Respiratory alkalosis	↑	↓	↓↓

Metabolic Acidosis

Anion Gap

P araldehyde
L actate
U remia
M ethanol
S alicylates
E thylene glycol
E thanol
D iabetic ketoacidosis

Non-anion Gap

D iarrhea, dilution
U reteral conduit
R enal tubular acidosis
H yperal
A cetazolamide, acid administration
M ultiple myeloma

As in Durham, N.C. home of the **Duke Blue Devils !!** *2001 NCAA Champions*

Metabolic Alkalosis

Chloride responsive
($U_{Cl} < 10$ mEq/L)
• GI losses (emesis, NG)
• diuretics
• chronic hypercapnea
• cystic fibrosis

Chloride resistant
($U_{Cl} > 10$ mEq/L)
• Cushing's syndrome
• Conn's syndrome
• exogenous steroids
• Barter's syndrome

GYN-ONCOLOGY

VIIA. ELECTROLYTE DISTURBANCES: HYPERKALEMIA

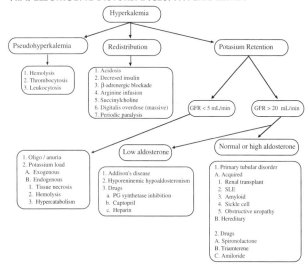

Treatment	Mechanism	Onset of Action
Calcium gluconate (10-30 mL of 10% solution)	Antagonize membrane effects	Few minutes
NaHCO₃ (44-132 Meq)	Redistribute	15-30 minutes
Glucose (50 g) and regular insulin (10 units)	Redistribute	15-30 minutes
Cation exchange resin (Kayexalate) Enema (50-100 g) Oral (40 g)	Remove	60 minutes 120 minutes
Dialysis Hemodialysis Peritoneal	Remove	Few minutes Few minutes

Source: Schrier RW. The patient with hypokalemia or hyperkalemia. In: Schrier RW, ed. *Manual of Nephrology: diagnosis and therapy.* 3rd ed. Boston: Little, Brown and Co, 1990. Reproduced with the permission of the publisher.

GYN-ONCOLOGY

B. HYPOKALEMIA

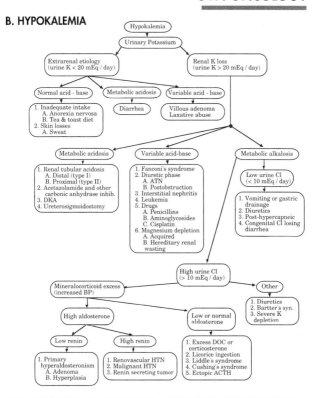

Source: Schrier RW. The patient with hypokalemia or hyperkalemia. In: Schrier RW, ed. *Manual of Nephrology: diagnosis and therapy.* 3rd ed. Boston: Little, Brown and Co, 1990. Reproduced with the permission of the publisher.

GYN-ONCOLOGY

C. HYPERCALCEMIA

Regulation of serum calcium

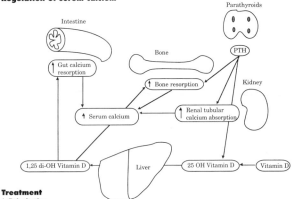

Treatment

1. Rehydration
- normal saline/half-normal saline
- furosemide 20 - 40 mg q 2 hr
- watch cardiac status, electrolytes

2. Glucocorticoids
- decrease intestinal absorption, bone remodeling, renal tubular absorption
- not useful in primary hyperparathyroidism
- hydrocortisone 250 - 500 mg IV q 8 hr
- may require several days

3. Calcitonin
- lowers calcium by 1-3 mg/dL for 6-8 hr
- skin test first
- starting dose 4 IU/kg SQ or IM q 12-24 hr
- use only if fluid/salt loading ineffective

4. Mithramycin
- toxic to osteoclasts
- useful in advanced malignancy
- dosing: 25 μg/kg by slow IV infusion q day
- calcium drops in 12 hr
- toxicity: thrombocytopenia, renal and hepatic damage

D. HYPONATREMIA

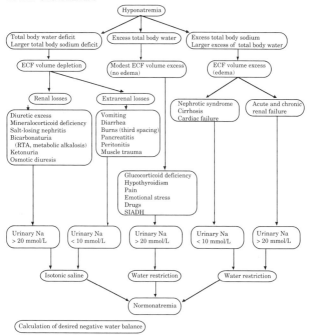

Calculation of desired negative water balance

Total Body Water (TBW) = Body Weight X 60%

$$\frac{\text{Actual Plasma Concentration}}{\text{Desired Plasma Concentration}} \times \text{TBW} = \text{Desired TBW}$$

Needed Neagative Water Balance = TBW - Desired TBW

Source: Schrier RW. The patient with hypokalemia or hyperkalemia. In: Schrier RW, ed. *Manual of Nephrology: diagnosis and therapy.* 3rd ed. Boston: Little, Brown and Co, 1990. Reproduced with the permission of the publisher.

GYN-ONCOLOGY

E. HYPERNATREMIA

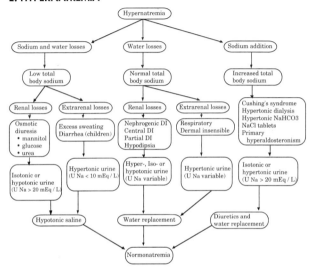

Hypernatremia

Sodium and water losses → Low total body sodium → Renal losses → Osmotic diuresis • mannitol • glucose • urea → Isotonic or hypotonic urine (U Na > 20 mEq / L) → Hypotonic saline

Extrarenal losses → Excess sweating Diarrhea (children) → Hypertonic urine (U Na < 10 mEq / L) → Hypotonic saline

Water losses → Normal total body sodium → Renal losses → Nephrogenic DI Central DI Partial DI Hypodipsia → Hyper-, Iso- or hypotonic urine (U Na variable) → Water replacement

Extrarenal losses → Respiratory Dermal insensible → Hypertonic urine (U Na variable) → Water replacement

Sodium addition → Increased total body sodium → Cushing's syndrome Hypertonic dialysis Hypertonic NaHCO3 NaCl tablets Primary hyperaldosteronism → Isotonic or hypertonic urine (U Na > 20 mEq / L) → Diuretics and water replacement

Normonatremia

Calculation of desired water replacement

Total Body Water (TBW) = Body Weight X 60%

$$\frac{\text{Actual Plasma Concentration}}{\text{Desired Plasma Concentration}} \times \text{TBW} = \text{Desired TBW}$$

Needed Positive Water Balance = Desired TBW - TBW

Source: Schrier RW. The patient with hypokalemia or hyperkalemia. In: Schrier RW, ed. *Manual of Nephrology: diagnosis and therapy.* 3rd ed. Boston: Little, Brown and Co, 1990. Reproduced with the permission of the publisher.

ACLS
ILCOR Universal Algorithm

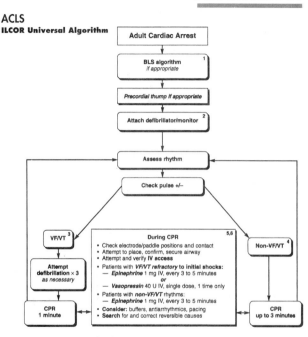

Source: Pages 211-225 are reproduced from The American Heart Association in collaboration with the International Liason Committee on Resuscitation (ILCOR). Guidelines 2000 for cardiopulmonary resuscitation and emergency cardiovascular care. *Circulation.* 2000;102(suppl I):I-142-I-157.

ACLS
Comprehensive ECC Algorithm

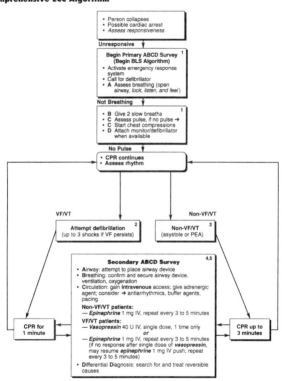

- Person collapses
- Possible cardiac arrest
- *Assess responsiveness*

Unresponsive ↓

Begin Primary ABCD Survey [1]
(Begin BLS Algorithm)
- Activate emergency response system
- Call for defibrillator
- **A** Assess breathing (open airway, *look, listen, and feel*)

Not Breathing ↓

- **B** Give 2 slow breaths [1]
- **C** Assess pulse, if no pulse →
- **C** Start chest compressions
- **D** Attach monitor/defibrillator when available

No Pulse ↓

- **CPR continues**
- **Assess rhythm**

VF/VT

Attempt defibrillation [2]
(up to 3 shocks if VF persists)

Non-VF/VT

Non-VF/VT [3]
(asystole or PEA)

Secondary ABCD Survey [4,5]
- Airway: attempt to place airway device
- Breathing: confirm and secure airway device, ventilation, oxygenation
- Circulation: gain **intravenous** access; give adrenergic agent; consider → antiarrhythmics, buffer agents, pacing

  Non-VF/VT patients:
  — *Epinephrine* 1 mg IV, repeat every 3 to 5 minutes

  VF/VT patients:
  — *Vasopressin* 40 U IV, single dose, 1 time only
     or
  — *Epinephrine* 1 mg IV, repeat every 3 to 5 minutes (if no response after single dose of *vasopressin*, may resume *epinephrine* 1 mg IV push; repeat every 3 to 5 minutes)

- Differential Diagnosis: search for and treat reversible causes

CPR for 1 minute

CPR up to 3 minutes

ACLS
Ventricular Fibrillation/Pulseless VT Algorithm

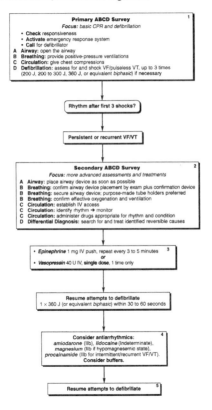

Primary ABCD Survey
Focus: basic CPR and defibrillation
- **Check** responsiveness
- **Activate** emergency response system
- **Call** for defibrillator
- A **Airway:** open the airway
- B **Breathing:** provide positive-pressure ventilations
- C **Circulation:** give chest compressions
- D **Defibrillation:** assess for and shock VF/pulseless VT, up to 3 times (200 J, 200 to 300 J, 360 J, or equivalent *biphasic*) if necessary

Rhythm after first 3 shocks?

Persistent or recurrent VF/VT

Secondary ABCD Survey
Focus: more advanced assessments and treatments
- A **Airway:** place airway device as soon as possible
- B **Breathing:** confirm airway device placement by exam plus confirmation device
- B **Breathing:** secure airway device; purpose-made tube holders preferred
- B **Breathing:** confirm effective oxygenation and ventilation
- C **Circulation:** establish IV access
- C **Circulation:** identify rhythm → monitor
- C **Circulation:** administer drugs appropriate for rhythm and condition
- D **Differential Diagnosis:** search for and treat identified reversible causes

- *Epinephrine* 1 mg IV push, repeat every 3 to 5 minutes
  or
- *Vasopressin* 40 U IV, **single dose,** 1 time only

Resume attempts to defibrillate
1 × 360 J (or equivalent *biphasic*) within 30 to 60 seconds

Consider antiarrhythmics:
amiodarone (IIb), *lidocaine* (Indeterminate), *magnesium* (IIb if hypomagnesemic state), *procainamide* (IIb for intermittent/recurrent VF/VT).
Consider buffers.

Resume attempts to defibrillate

GYN-ONCOLOGY

ACLS
Pulseless Electrical Activity Algorithm

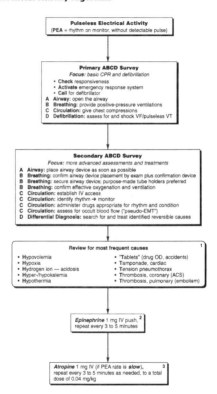

Pulseless Electrical Activity
(PEA = rhythm on monitor, without detectable pulse)

Primary ABCD Survey
Focus: basic CPR and defibrillation
- Check responsiveness
- Activate emergency response system
- Call for defibrillator
A **Airway:** open the airway
B **Breathing:** provide positive-pressure ventilations
C **Circulation:** give chest compressions
D **Defibrillation:** assess for and shock VF/pulseless VT

Secondary ABCD Survey
Focus: more advanced assessments and treatments
A **Airway:** place airway device as soon as possible
B **Breathing:** confirm airway device placement by exam plus confirmation device
B **Breathing:** secure airway device; purpose-made tube holders preferred
B **Breathing:** confirm effective oxygenation and ventilation
C **Circulation:** establish IV access
C **Circulation:** identify rhythm → monitor
C **Circulation:** administer drugs appropriate for rhythm and condition
C **Circulation:** assess for occult blood flow ("pseudo-EMT")
D **Differential Diagnosis:** search for and treat identified reversible causes

Review for most frequent causes [1]
- Hypovolemia
- Hypoxia
- Hydrogen ion — acidosis
- Hyper-/hypokalemia
- Hypothermia
- "Tablets" (drug OD, accidents)
- Tamponade, cardiac
- Tension pneumothorax
- Thrombosis, coronary (ACS)
- Thrombosis, pulmonary (embolism)

Epinephrine 1 mg IV push, [2]
repeat every 3 to 5 minutes

Atropine 1 mg IV (if PEA rate is *slow*), [3]
repeat every 3 to 5 minutes as needed, to a total
dose of 0.04 mg/kg

ACLS
Asystole: The Silent Heart Algorithm

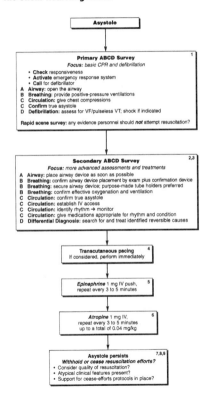

Asystole

Primary ABCD Survey [1]
Focus: basic CPR and defibrillation

- **Check** responsiveness
- **Activate** emergency response system
- **Call** for defibrillator

A **Airway:** open the airway
B **Breathing:** provide positive-pressure ventilations
C **Circulation:** give chest compressions
C **Confirm** true asystole
D **Defibrillation:** assess for VF/pulseless VT; shock if indicated

Rapid scene survey: any evidence personnel should *not* attempt resuscitation?

Secondary ABCD Survey [2,3]
Focus: more advanced assessments and treatments

A **Airway:** place airway device as soon as possible
B **Breathing:** confirm airway device placement by exam plus confirmation device
B **Breathing:** secure airway device; purpose-made tube holders preferred
B **Breathing:** confirm effective oxygenation and ventilation
C **Circulation:** confirm true asystole
C **Circulation:** establish IV access
C **Circulation:** identify rhythm → monitor
C **Circulation:** give medications appropriate for rhythm and condition
D **Differential Diagnosis:** search for and treat identified reversible causes

Transcutaneous pacing [4]
If considered, perform immediately

Epinephrine 1 mg IV push, [5]
repeat every 3 to 5 minutes

Atropine 1 mg IV, [6]
repeat every 3 to 5 minutes
up to a total of 0.04 mg/kg

Asystole persists [7,8,9]
Withhold or cease resuscitation efforts?
- Consider quality of resuscitation?
- Atypical clinical features present?
- Support for cease-efforts protocols in place?

ACLS
Bradycardia Algorithm

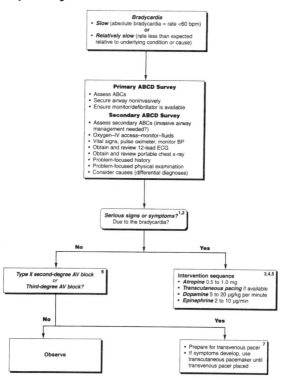

Bradycardia
- *Slow* (absolute bradycardia = rate <60 bpm)

or

- *Relatively slow* (rate less than expected relative to underlying condition or cause)

Primary ABCD Survey
- Assess ABCs
- Secure airway noninvasively
- Ensure monitor/defibrillator is available

Secondary ABCD Survey
- Assess secondary ABCs (invasive airway management needed?)
- Oxygen–IV access–monitor–fluids
- Vital signs, pulse oximeter, monitor BP
- Obtain and review 12-lead ECG
- Obtain and review portable chest x-ray
- Problem-focused history
- Problem-focused physical examination
- Consider causes (differential diagnoses)

Serious signs or symptoms?[1,2]
Due to the bradycardia?

No

Yes

Type II second-degree AV block[6]

or

Third-degree AV block?

Intervention sequence [3,4,5]
- *Atropine* 0.5 to 1.0 mg
- *Transcutaneous pacing* if available
- *Dopamine* 5 to 20 µg/kg per minute
- *Epinephrine* 2 to 10 µg/min

No

Yes

Observe

- Prepare for transvenous pacer[7]
- If symptoms develop, use transcutaneous pacemaker until transvenous pacer placed

ACLS
Tachycardia Overview Algorithm

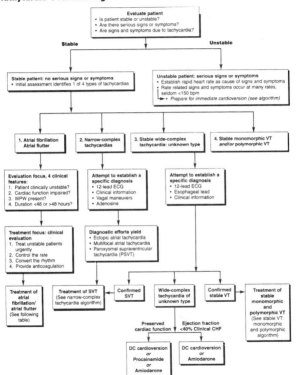

GYN-ONCOLOGY

ACLS
Tachycardia Overview

Control of Rate and Rhythm (Continued From Tachycardia Overview)

Atrial fibrillation/ atrial flutter with • Normal heart • Impaired heart • WPW	1. Control Rate		2. Convert Rhythm	
	Heart Function Preserved	Impaired Heart EF <40% or CHF	Duration <48 Hours	Duration >48 Hours or Unknown
Normal cardiac function	Note: If AF >48 hours' duration, use agents to convert rhythm with extreme caution in patients not receiving adequate anticoagulation because of possible embolic complications. Use only 1 of the following agents (see note below): • Calcium channel blockers (Class I) • β-Blockers (Class I) • For additional drugs that are Class IIb recommendations, see Guidelines or ACLS text	(Does not apply)	Consider • DC cardioversion Use only 1 of the following agents (see note below): • Amiodarone (Class IIa) • Ibutilide (Class IIa) • Flecainide (Class IIa) • Propafenone (Class IIa) • Procainamide (Class IIa) • For additional drugs that are Class IIb recommendations, see Guidelines or ACLS text	• NO DC cardioversion! • Note: Conversion of AF to NSR with drugs or shock may cause embolization of atrial thrombi unless patient has adequate anticoagulation. • Use antiarrhythmic agents with extreme caution if AF >48 hours' duration (see note above). or Delayed cardioversion Anticoagulation × 3 weeks at proper levels • Cardioversion, then • Anticoagulation × 4 weeks more or Early cardioversion • Begin IV heparin at once • TEE to exclude atrial clot then • Cardioversion within 24 hours then • Anticoagulation × 4 more weeks
Impaired heart (EF <40% or CHF)	(Does not apply)	Note: If AF >48 hours' duration, use agents to convert rhythm with extreme caution in patients not receiving adequate anticoagulation because of possible embolic complications. Use only 1 of the following agents (see note below): • Digoxin (Class IIb) • Diltiazem (Class IIb) • Amiodarone (Class IIb)	Consider • DC cardioversion or • Amiodarone (Class IIb)	• Anticoagulation as described above, followed by • DC cardioversion

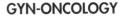
ACLS
Tachycardia Overview

Control of Rate and Rhythm (Continued From Tachycardia Overview)

Atrial fibrillation/ atrial flutter with • Normal heart • Impaired heart • WPW	1. Control Rate		2. Convert Rhythm	
	Heart Function Preserved	Impaired Heart EF <40% or CHF	Duration <48 Hours	Duration >48 Hours or Unknown

WPW	**Note:** *If AF >48 hours' duration, use agents to convert rhythm with extreme caution in patients not receiving adequate anticoagulation because of possible embolic complications.*
	
	• DC cardioversion
	  or
	• **Primary anti-arrhythmic agents** Use only 1 of the following agents (see note below):
	• Amiodarone (Class IIb)
	• Flecainide (Class IIb)
	• Procainamide (Class IIb)
	• Propafenone (Class IIb)
	• Sotalol (Class IIb)
	
	Class III (can be harmful)
	• Adenosine
	• β-Blockers
	• Calcium blockers
	• Digoxin
		Note: *If AF >48 hours' duration. use agents to convert rhythm with extreme caution in patients not receiving adequate anticoagulation because of possible embolic complications.*
		
		• DC cardioversion
		  or
		• Amiodarone (Class IIb)
			• DC cardioversion
			  or
			• **Primary anti-arrhythmic agents** Use only 1 of the following agents (see note below**):
			• Amiodarone (Class IIb)
			• Flecainide (Class IIb)
			• Procainamide (Class IIb)
			• Propafenone (Class IIb)
			• Sotalol (Class IIb)
			
			Class III (can be harmful)
			• Adenosine
			• β-Blockers
			• Calcium blockers
			• Digoxin
				• **Anticoagulation** as described above, followed by
				• **DC cardioversion**

WPW indicates Wolff-Parkinson-White syndrome; AF, atrial fibrillation; NSR, normal sinus rhythm; TEE, transesophageal echocardiogram; and EF, ejection fraction.

Note: Occasionally 2 of the named antiarrhythmic agents may be used, but use of these agents in combination may have proarrhythmic potential. The classes listed represent the Class of Recommendation rather than the Vaughn-Williams classification of antiarrhythmics.

GYN-ONCOLOGY

ACLS
Narrow-Complex Supraventricular Tachycardia Algorithm

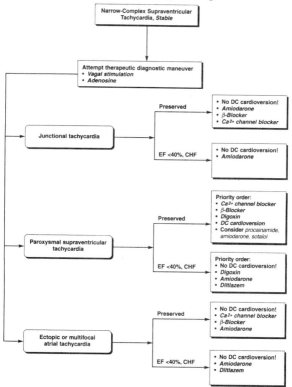

ACLS
Stable Ventricular Tachycardia (Monomorphic or Polymorphic Algorithm)

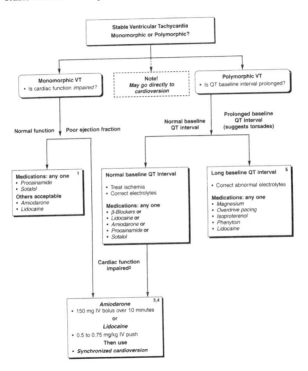

GYN-ONCOLOGY

ACLS
Synchronized Cardioversion Algorithm

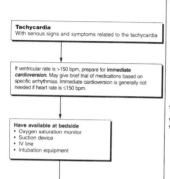

Tachycardia
With serious signs and symptoms related to the tachycardia

If ventricular rate is >150 bpm, prepare for **immediate cardioversion**. May give brief trial of medications based on specific arrhythmias. Immediate cardioversion is generally not needed if heart rate is ≤150 bpm.

Have available at bedside
• Oxygen saturation monitor
• Suction device
• IV line
• Intubation equipment

Premediate whenever possible ¹

Synchronized cardioversion 2,3,4,5,6
• Ventricular tachycardia
• Paroxysmal supraventricular tachycardia
• Atrial fibrillation
• Atrial flutter

100 J, 200 J,
300 J, 360 J
monophasic energy
dose (or clinically
equivalent biphasic
energy dose)

Steps for
Synchronized Cardioversion

1. Consider sedation.
2. Turn on defibrillator (monophasic or biphasic).
3. Attach monitor leads to the patient ("white to right, red to ribs, what's left over to the left shoulder") and ensure proper display of the patient's rhythm.
4. Engage the synchronization mode by pressing the "sync" control button.
5. Look for markers on R waves indicating sync mode.
6. If necessary, adjust monitor gain until sync markers occur with each R wave.
7. Select appropriate energy level.
8. Position conductor pads on patient (or apply gel to paddles).
9. Position paddle on patient (sternum-apex).
10. Announce to team members:
   "Charging defibrillator—stand clear!"
11. Press "charge" button on apex paddle (right hand).
12. When the defibrillator is charged, begin the final clearing chant. State firmly in a forceful voice the following chant before each shock:
   • "I am going to shock on three. One, I'm clear." (Check to make sure you are clear of contact with the patient, the stretcher, and the equipment.)
   • "Two, you are clear." (Make a visual check to ensure that no one continues to touch the patient or stretcher. In particular, do not forget about the person providing ventilations. That person's hands should not be touching the ventilatory adjuncts, including the tracheal tube!)
   • "Three, everybody's clear." (Check yourself one more time before pressing the "shock" buttons.)
13. Apply 25 lb pressure on both paddles.
14. Press the "discharge" buttons simultaneously.
15. Check the monitor. If tachycardia persists, increase the joules according to the electrical cardioversion algorithm.
16. Reset the sync mode after each synchronized cardioversion because most defibrillators default back to unsynchronized mode. This default allows an immediate defibrillation if the cardioversion produces VF.

Notes:
1. Effective regimens have included a sedative (eg. *diazepam, midazolam, barbiturates, etomidate, ketamine, methohexital*) with or without an analgesic agent (eg, *fentanyl, morphine, meperidine*). Many experts recommend anesthesia if service is readily available.
2. Both monophasic and biphasic waveforms are acceptable if documented as clinically equivalent to reports of monophasic shock success.
3. Note possible need to resynchronize after each cardioversion.
4. If delays in synchronization occur and clinical condition is critical, go immediately to unsynchronized shocks.
5. Treat polymorphic ventricular tachycardia (irregular form and rate) like ventricular fibrillation: see ventricular fibrillation/pulseless ventricular tachycardia algorithm.
6. Paroxysmal supraventricular tachycardia and atrial flutter often respond to lower energy levels (start with 50 J).

ACLS
Acute Ischemic Chest Pain Algorithm

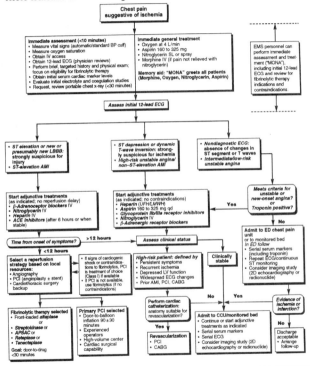

This algorithm provides general guidelines that may not apply to all patients. Carefully consider proper indications and contraindications.

GYN-ONCOLOGY

ACLS
Acute Coronary Syndromes Algorithm

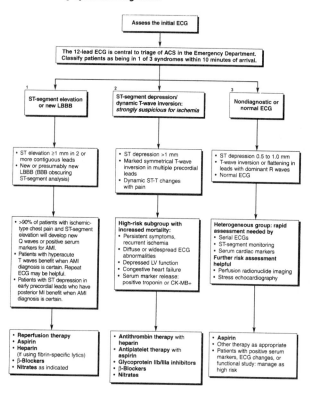

```
                    ┌──────────────────────────┐
                    │   Assess the initial ECG │
                    └──────────────────────────┘

┌─────────────────────────────────────────────────────────────────┐
│ The 12-lead ECG is central to triage of ACS in the Emergency     │
│ Department. Classify patients as being in 1 of 3 syndromes        │
│ within 10 minutes of arrival.                                     │
└─────────────────────────────────────────────────────────────────┘
```

1
ST-segment elevation or new LBBB

- ST elevation ≥1 mm in 2 or more contiguous leads
- New or presumably new LBBB (BBB obscuring ST-segment analysis)

- >90% of patients with ischemic-type chest pain and ST-segment elevation will develop new Q waves or positive serum markers for AMI.
- Patients with hyperacute T waves benefit when AMI diagnosis is certain. Repeat ECG may be helpful.
- Patients with ST depression in early precordial leads who have posterior MI benefit when AMI diagnosis is certain.

- **Reperfusion therapy**
- **Aspirin**
- **Heparin** (if using fibrin-specific lytics)
- **β-Blockers**
- **Nitrates** as indicated

2
ST-segment depression/ dynamic T-wave inversion: *strongly suspicious for ischemia*

- ST depression >1 mm
- Marked symmetrical T-wave inversion in multiple precordial leads
- Dynamic ST-T changes with pain

High-risk subgroup with increased mortality:
- Persistent symptoms, recurrent ischemia
- Diffuse or widespread ECG abnormalities
- Depressed LV function
- Congestive heart failure
- Serum marker release: positive troponin or CK-MB+

- **Antithrombin therapy with heparin**
- **Antiplatelet therapy with aspirin**
- **Glycoprotein IIb/IIIa inhibitors**
- **β-Blockers**
- **Nitrates**

3
Nondiagnostic or normal ECG

- ST depression 0.5 to 1.0 mm
- T-wave inversion or flattening in leads with dominant R waves
- Normal ECG

Heterogeneous group: rapid assessment needed by
- Serial ECGs
- ST-segment monitoring
- Serum cardiac markers
Further risk assessment helpful
- Perfusion radionuclide imaging
- Stress echocardiography

- **Aspirin**
- Other therapy as appropriate
- Patients with positive serum markers, ECG changes, or functional study: manage as high risk

ACLS
Acute Pulmonary Edema, Hypotension, and Shock Algorithm

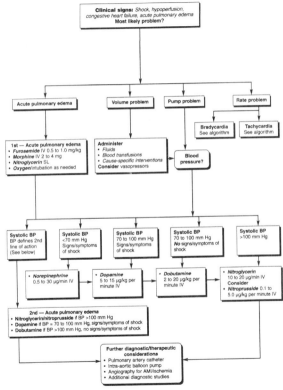

233

ENDOCRINOLOGY

MENSTRUAL CYCLE

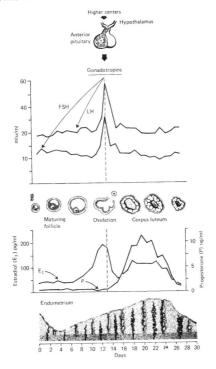

Source: Couchman GM, Hammond CB. Physiology of reproduction. In: Scott JR, DiSaia PD, Hammond CB, Spellacy WN, ed. *Danforth's Obstetrics and Gynecology.* 7th ed. Philadelphia: Lippincott, 1994. Reproduced with the permission of the publisher.

ENDOCRINOLOGY

WHO CLASSIFICATION OF OVARIAN INSUFFICIENCY

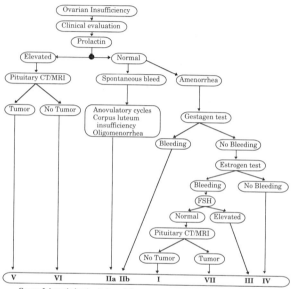

Group I: hypothalamic pituitary failure
Group II: hypothalamic pituitary dysfunction
Group III: ovarian failure
Group IV: congenital or acquired genital tract disorders
Group V: hyperprolactinemic infertile women with pituitary tumor
Group VI: hyperprolactinemic infertile women without detectable pituitary tumor
Group VII: normoprolactinemic amenorrhea and lesion in hypothal-pituitary region

ENDOCRINOLOGY

DISORDERS OF PUBERTY
Precocious Puberty

Classification	Female	Male	puberty
GnRH independent (True Precocity)			
Idiopathic	74%	41%	
CNS problem	7%	26%	
GnRH Independent (Precocious Psuedopuberty)			
Ovarian (cyst or tumor)	11%	-	
Testicular	-	10%	
McCune-Albright syndrome	5%	1%	
Adrenal feminizing	1%	0%	
Adrenal masculinizing	1%	22%	
Ectopic gonadotropin production	0.5%	0.5%	

Relative Frequency of Delayed Pubertal Abnormalities

Classification		
Hypergonadotropic hypogonadism	43%	
Ovarian failure, abnormal karyotype	26%	
Ovarian failure, normal karyotype	17%	
46, XX		15%
46, XY		2%
Hypogonadotropic hypogonadism	31%	
Reversible	18%	
Physiologic delay		10%
Weight loss/anorexia		3%
Primary hypothyroidism		1%
Congenital adrenal hyperplasia		1%
Cushing's syndrome		0.5%
Prolactinomas		1.5%
Irreversible	13%	
GnRH deficiency		7%
Hypopituitarism		2%
Congenital CNS defects		0.5%
Other pituitary adenomas		0.5%
Craniopharyngioma		1%
Malignant pituitary tumor		0.5%
Eugonadism	26%	
Müllerian agenesis		14%
Vaginal septum		3%
Imperforate hymen		0.5%
Androgen insensitivity syndrome		1%
Inappropriate positive feedback		7%

Source: Speroff L, Glass RH, Kase NG. Abnormal puberty and growth problems. In: *Clinical Gynecologic Endocrinology and Infertility*. 6th ed. Philadelphia: Lippincott Williams & Wilkins, 1999. Reproduced with the permission of the publisher.

ENDOCRINOLOGY

AMENORRHEA

Definition
• no menses by age 14 in absence of 2° sexual characteristics (primary)
• no menses by age 16 despite 2° sexual characteristics (primary)
• no menses in 6 months (secondary)

Etiology
Primary
43% Gonadal failure
15% Congenital absence of the vagina
14% Constitutional delay

Secondary
39% Chronic anovulation
20% Hypothyroidism/hyperprolactinemia
16% Weight loss/anorexia

Vaginal Agenesis vs. Androgen Insensitivity Syndrome

	Mayer-Rokitansky-Kuster-Hauser Syndrome	Complete Androgen Insensitivity Syndrome
Vagina	absent	absent
Pubic hair	present	absent
Breasts	present	present
Gonads	ovaries	testes
Uterus	absent	absent
Karyotype	46, XX	46, XY
Other anomalies (renal, cardiac)	increased	not increased

AMENORRHEA
Diagnostic Algorithm

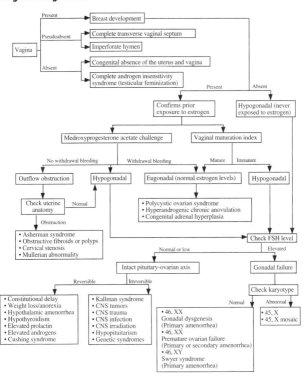

Source: Penzias AS. A basic guide to evaluating amenorrhea. *The Female Patient* 1999;24:57-62. Reproduced with permission.

239

ENDOCRINOLOGY

STEROID BIOSYNTHESIS

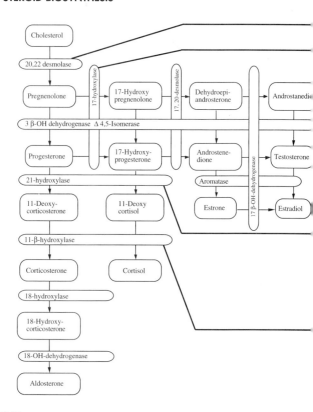

20-22 Desmolase Deficiency (adrenal and ovary)
- lethal
- internal/external female genitalia
- adrenal enlarged with cholesterol esters

17 α-Hydroxylase Deficiency (adrenal and ovary)
- hypertension, hypokalemia
- infantile female external genitalia
- primary amenorrhea with elevated FSH and LH
- genital ambiguity in male infants only

3 β-Hydroxysteroid Dehydrogenase Deficiency (adrenal and ovary)
- infants severely ill at birth
- rarely survive
- females slightly virilized, males incompletely masculinized
- milder non-classic cases may be common

21-Hydroxylase Deficiency (adrenal only)
- most common form of congenital adrenal hyperplasia (>90%)
- most frequent cause of sexual ambiguity
- most frequent endocrine cause of neonatal death
  - salt-wasting
  - hypertension
- 3 clinical forms
  - salt-wasting (cortisol and aldosterone)
  - simple virilizing (cortisol production only)
  - late-onset
- inherited as monogenic autosomal recessive
  - close linkage to HLA complex on short arm of chromosome 6
- diagnosis by increased 17-OHP (baseline or with ACTH stim. test)

11 β-Hydroxylase Deficiency (adrenal only)
- 11-deoxycortisol not converted to cortisol
- desoxycorticosterone not converted to corticosterone
- variable affect on aldosterone levels
- hypertension, hypokalemia (usually mild after several years of life)
- diagnosis by high levels of DOC and compound S (11-deoxycortisol)

Source: Speroff L, Glass RH, Kase NG. Normal and abnormal sexual development. In: *Clinical Gynecologic Endocrinology and Infertility.* 6th ed. Philadelphia: Lippincott Williams & Wilkins, 1999. Reproduced with the permission of the publisher.

ENDOCRINOLOGY

POLYCYSTIC OVARIAN SYNDROME (PCOS)

Fast Facts
• originally described by Stein & Leventhal 1935
• endocrine imbalance involving hypothalamic-pituitary-ovarian-adrenal axis

Clinical Symptoms
• menstrual disorders (80%)
• hirsutism (69%)
• obesity (49%)
• infertility (74%)

Ovarian Morphology
• bilateral enlargement
• multiple small follicles with thick ovarian capsule
• follicles in various stages of growth/atresia
• hyperthecosis (luteinization of theca interna/reduction of granulosa cells)

Hormonal Status
• elevated LH/FSH ratio (>2.0) in most patients
• exaggerated pulsatile LH levels
• increased androgens (androstenedione, testosterone)
• decreased SHBG (increased free testosterone)

Medical Therapy
• clomiphene citrate (CC, Serophene): mainly for ovulatory dysfunction
• gonadotropins (FSH/LH; Metrodin, Pergonal): following CC failure, beware of OHSS
• pure FSH/hCG (Metrodin, Profasi): probably more efficient than hMG
• glucocorticoids (prednisone, dexamethasone): particularly in cases of adult onset
  adrenocortical hyperplasia and clinical findings of PCO
• dopamine agonists (bromocriptine): if associated with hyperprolactinemia

Surgical Therapy
• ovarian wedge resection
  • 80% will resume normal cycles
  • 63% will conceive
  • may result in pertubular and ovarian adhesions
• laparoscopic ovarian drilling
  • results may be similar to wedge resection
  • may be minimally invasive option for medical failures

Assisted Reproductive Technologies
• results similar to other groups except "mechanical infertility"
• beware of OHSS

POLYCYSTIC OVARIAN SYNDROME (PCOS)
Pathophysiology

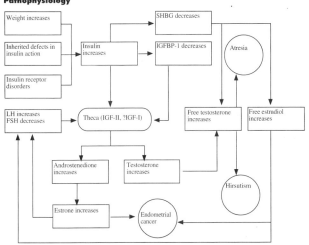

Source: Speroff L, Glass RH, Kase NG. Anovulation and the polycystic ovary. In: *Clinical Gynecologic Endocrinology and Infertility.* 6th ed. Philadelphia: Lippincott Williams & Wilkins, 1999. Reproduced with the permission of the publisher.

Insulin Resistance
• increasing body of evidence linking insulin resistance and PCOS
• all patients with PCOS should be assessed with a fasting glucose:insulin ratio and a 2 hr 75 g GTT
    • fasting glucose:insulin ratio <4.5 is consistent with insulin resistance
    • 2 hr GTT should be < 140 mg/dL; 140-199 mg/dL represents impaired glucose tolerance
        • 2 hr GTT > 200 mg/dL represents noninsulin-dependent diabetes mellitus
• treatment with insulin sensitizing agents such as metformin may improve response to ovulation
    induction and recent data also suggests it may decrease first trimester spontaneous abortion
        • GI distress is common with metformin, especially at doses of 500 mg tid

ENDOCRINOLOGY

HIRSUTISM
Fast Facts
• Definition: male type body hair distribution (sexual hair areas)
  • face - mustache, beard, sideburns
  • body - chest, circumareolar, linea alba, abdominal trigone, inner thighs
• 1/3 of women age 14-45 have excessive upper lip hair
• 6-9% have unwanted chin/sideburn hair
• Cushing's Syndrome
  • most common referral diagnosis, one of the least common final diagnoses
• hair follicles laid down at 8 weeks gestation
• cyclic hair growth
  • anagen: growing phase
  • catagen: rapid involution phase
  • telogen: resting phase

Differential Diagnosis
Hypertrichosis
a. drugs: phenytoin, streptomycin, steroids, penicillamine, diazoxide, minoxidil
b. pathologic states: hypothyroidism, anorexia, dermatomyositis, porphyria
c. normal states: older age, ethnic background, pregnancy

Hirsutism (increase in sexual hair)
Endogenous androgen overproduction
Tumors
Adrenal: adrenocortical tumors, adenomas, carcinomas
Ovarian: arrhenoblastomas, hilar cell, Krukenberg
Pituitary: adenomas

Non-tumors
Adrenal: congenital adrenal hyperplasia
• 21-hydroxylase deficiency
• 11-hydroxylase deficiency
Cushing's Syndrome

Ovary: androgenized ovary syndrome
• polycystic ovaries
• hyperthecosis

Initial Laboratory Studies
• testosterone (> 200 ng/dL possible adrenal tumor)
• DHAS (> 700 µg/dL adrenal hyperplasia or tumor)
• 17-OH progesterone (< 300 ng/dL or suppressible rules out adrenal hyperplasia)
• prolactin
• TSH
• endometrial biopsy (individualize)

HIRSUTISM

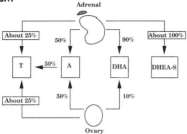

Source: Speroff L, Glass RH, Kase NG. Hirsutism. In: *Clinical Gynecologic Endocrinology and Infertility*. 6th ed. Philadelphia:Lippincott Williams & Wilkins, 1999. Reproduced with the permission of the publisher.

Treatment

- almost all patients represent excessive androgen production from anovulatory ovary
- treatment aims at interrupting one or more steps in pathway to DHT

  Inhibition of adrenal or ovarian androgen secretion
  Alteration of binding androgens to SHBG
  Impairment of the peripheral conversion of androgen precursors to active androgens
  Inhibition of androgen action at the target tissue

Options
- combination OCP's (Demulen)
- Depo-Provera 150 mg IM q 3 months
- medroxyprogesterone acetate (Provera) 30 mg q day
- spironolactone 200 mg q day (need to also use contraception)
- GnRH-agonists
- finasteride (must avoid pregnancy)
- flutamide (risk of liver toxicity)

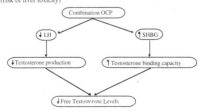

ENDOCRINOLOGY

HYPERPROLACTINEMIA

Fast Facts

- polypeptide hormone with 198 amino acids produced in anterior pituitary
- resembles human growth hormone (hCG) and human placental lactogen (hPL)
- production is under tonic control of prolactin inhibiting factor (PIF) probably dopamine
- thyroid releasing hormone (TRH) is potent stimulant
- normal levels 5-25 ng/mL in adult women
- may present as galactorrhea, amenorrhea, or infertility

Evaluation

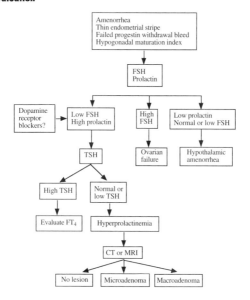

Source: Faber KA. A pragmatic approach to evaluating, managing hyperprolactinemia. *OBG Management* 1998; June:66-79. Reproduced with permission.

HYPERPROLACTINEMIA

Etiology

Physiologic Causes
Breast stimulation or suckling
Coitus
Eating
Exercise
Pregnancy
Puerperium
Sleep
Stress

Non-neoplastic Causes
Afferent neural stimulation
  • breast
      • chronic abscess
      • excessive manipulation
  • chest wall and skin
      • herpes zoster
      • mastectomy
      • thoracotomy
  • spinal cord
      • syringomyelia
      • tabes dorsalis
Endocrine function
  • adrenal tumors
  • hypothyroidism
  • ovarian tumors
  • polycystic ovary disease
Inhibition of PIF synthesis
  • hypothalamic
  • infarction
  • infiltrative disease
      • encephalitis or postencephalitis
      • hemochromatosis
      • sarcoidosis
      • Schuller-Christian disease
  • irradiation
  • pseudocyesis
  • Parkinson's disease
Interruption of PIF transport
  • pituitary stalk section
  • pituitary stalk compression
      • aneurysm
      • cysts
      • empty sella syndrome
      • pseudotumor cerebri
Other
  • acute intermittent porphyria
  • hepatic cirrhosis
  • renal failure

Pharmacological Causes
Amphetamines
Antihypertensives
      • reserpine
      • alpha methyldopa
Dopamine antagonists
      • metoclopramide
Opioides
Steroids
      • danazol
      • estrogen
      • medroxyprogesterone acetate
      • oral contraceptive
Tranquilizers
      • butyrophenones
      • phenothiazines
      • thioxanthenes
      • tricyclic antidepressants
Other
      • cimetidine
      • general anesthesia
      • isoniazid

Neoplastic Causes
Inhibition of PIF synthesis
  • hypothalamic tumors
      • primary (e.g. craniopharyngioma)
      • metastatic
  • pineal tumors
      • primary
      • metastatic
Interruption of PIF transport
  • pituitary stalk compression
      • hypothalamic tumors
      • pituitary tumors
Prolactin-secreting tumors
  • pituitary tumors
      • acromegaly
      • Cushing's disease
      • Nelson's disease
      • prolactin secreting
        (micro-or macro adenoma)
  • ectopic tumor production
      • breast carcinoma
      • bronchogenic carcinoma
      • hyperephroma

Source: Maxson WS, Hammond CB. Hyperprolactinemia-the underlying physiology. *Cont Ob/Gyn* 1982;19(1):49. Reproduced with the permission of the publisher, Medical Economics Publishing.

ENDOCRINOLOGY

HYPERPROLACTINEMIA
Treatment

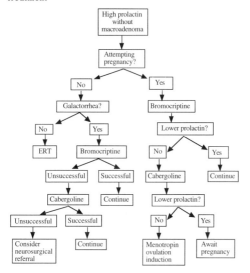

Source: Faber KA. A pragmatic approach to evaluating, managing hyperprolactinemia. *OBG Management* 1998; June:66-79. Reproduced with permission.

THYROID DISEASE
Fast Facts
• thyroid dysfunction is very common with 13 million Americans with some sort of thyroid disorder
• hypothyroidism occurs in 2% of adults and subclinical hypothyroidism in 5-17%
• early treatment of subclinical hypothyroidism may improve pregnancy outcome

Common Symptoms
Hyperthyroidism
Anxiousness
Tremulousness
Rapid heartbeat
Feeling of warmth
Difficulty concentrating
Muscle weakness
Weight loss

Hypothyroidism
Fatigue
Weakness
Weight gain
Constipation
Memory impairment
Cold intolerance
Muscle cramps

Differential Diagnosis of Low TSH During First Trimester
Subclinical hyperthyroidism
• 15% of normal pregnancies
• multiple gestation
• mild nausea, vomiting
• iatrogenic (thyroid therapy)

Hyperthyroidism
• multiple gestation
• transient thyrotoxicosis
• hyperemesis gravidarum
• Graves' disease
• iatrogenic (thyroid therapy)

ENDOCRINOLOGY

THYROID DISEASE
Evaluation

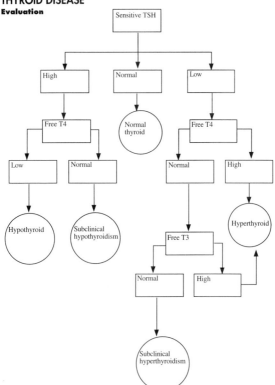

THYROID DISEASE
Etiologies

Primary hypothyroidism	Central hypothyroidism
Autoimmune thyroiditis (Hashimoto's)	**Hypothalamic/pituitary disease**
Postthyroidectomy	Tumors
Postradioactive iodine ablation	Infiltative diseases
Abnormal thyroid hormone biosynthesis	Radiation therapy
Iodine deficiency	Postpartum pituitary necrosis
Inherited enzyme defects	Lymphocytic hypophysitis
Antithyroid drugs	Head trauma
Thyroiditis (transient)	
Silent thyroiditis	
Subacute thyroiditis	
Postpartum thyroiditis	
Infiltrative thyroid diseases	
Sarcoid	
Amyloidosis	
Hemochromatosis	

Primary hyperthyroidism	Central hyperthyroidism
High radionuclide uptake	**High radionuclide uptake**
Graves' disease	TSH-secreting pituitary adenoma
Toxic nodular goiter*	Thyroid hormone resistance
Toxic nodule*	
HCG-induced hyperthyroidism	
Low radionuclide uptake	
Thyroiditis (transient)	
Silent thyroiditis	
Subacute thyroiditis	
Postpartum thyroiditis	
Excessive thyroid hormone	
Ectopic thyroid tissue (struma ovarii)	

*Radionuclide uptake may be within normal range

Source: Mulder JE. Thyroid disease in women. *Med Clin North Am* 1998;82(1):103-125.

INFERTILITY

BASIC INFERTILITY
Fast Facts
• 15% of all couples have infertility
• female factor 40% (ovulation, pelvis/tubes, uterus, cervix)
• male factor 40%
• unexplained 20%
• fecundity naturally 20% each cycle, 50% at 3 months, 85% at 1 year

Evaluation

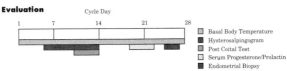

Cycle Day

1	7	14	21	28

◻ Basal Body Temperature
◻ Hysterosalpingogram
◻ Post Coital Test
◻ Serum Progesterone/Prolactin
◼ Endometrial Biopsy

Semen Analysis (SA)
• abstain 2 day prior
• deliver to lab in 2 hr
• if poor SA -> repeat 3 weeks
• still poor -> Andrologist

Consistency	Fluid (after liquefaction)
Color	Opaque
Liquefaction Time	20-30 minutes
pH	7.2-7.8
Volume	2-5 ml
Motility	> 30% (progressive)
Motility	50% (total)
Count	20-250 million/mL
Morphology	50% oval form
Cells	None
Mean Velocity	25 μm/s
Progression	50%

Post Coital Test (PCT)
• done after semen analysis
• look at mid cycle and determine time of ovulation
• abstain 2 days
• perform test 1-2 day before ovulation
• perform test 2-12 hr after coitus
• Spinnbarkheit 6 cm
• 10^5 motile (forward) sperm/hpf
• pH 6
• few wbc
• increased wbc; treat with antibiotics
• shaky sperm; antisperm antibodies

Basal Body Temperature (BBT)
• test to confirm ovulation
• oral temperature q AM before arising
    • should rise 0.4-0.6° C > 10 days

Endometrial Biopsy (EMBx)
Proliferative phase
• early (CD 4-7): scant narrow glands
• mid (CD 8-10): long curving glands with freq. mitoses
• late (CD 11-14): tortuous glands and undulating surface epithelium

Secretory phase
• ovulation + 2: subnuclear vacuoles
• ovulation + 6: peak intraluminal secretions
• ovulation + 7: beginning stromal edema
• ovulation + 8: maximum stromal edema
• ovulation + 10: periarteriolar predecidualization
• ovulation + 11: subsurface predecidualization
• ovulation + 12: coalescence of islands of predecidua
• ovulation + 13: confluence of predecidualization
• ovulation + 14: extravasation of rbc's in stroma

INFERTILITY

EVALUATION OF THE AZOOSPERMIC MALE

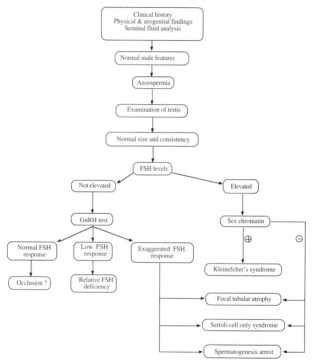

Source: Glezerman, M. and Lunenfeld B. Diagnosis of male infertility. In: Insler V, Lunenfeld B, ed. *Infertility: Male and Female.* 2nd ed. Edinburgh New York: Churchill Livingstone, 1993. Reproduced with the permission of the publisher.

EJACULATORY FAILURE

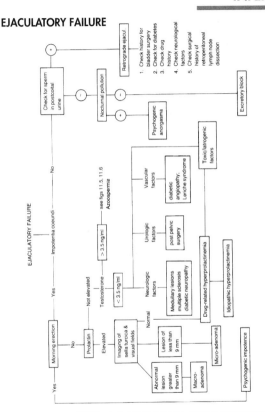

Source: Glezerman, M. and Lunenfeld B. Diagnosis of male infertility. In: Insler V, Lunenfeld B, ed. *Infertility: Male and Female.* 2nd ed. Edinburgh, New York: Churchill Livingstone, 1993. Reproduced with the permission of the publisher.

INFERTILITY

OVULATION INDUCTION

Fast Facts
• anovulation and ovulatory disorders present in 20% of infertile couples
• ovulation can be achieved in > 90% and 50-70% will conceive
• rule out other etiologies of anovulation prior to therapy
    • ovarian failure (gonadal dysgenesis, premature ovarian failure) - FSH level
    • adrenal disorders (Addison's, Cushing's, congenital adrenal hyperplasia)
    • thyroid dysfunction
• evaluate prolactin, TSH, progestin withdrawl bleed, semen analysis

Clomiphene Citrate (Serophene, Clomid)
• weak estrogen that functions as anti-estrogen
• requires intact hypothalamic-pituitary-ovarian axis

    "Rule of five 5's"
        • oral progestin 10 mg q day x 5 days (after negative ß-hCG)
        • begin clomiphene on day 5 of bleeding
        • 50 mg clomiphene q day x 5 days
        • timed coitus 5 days later and for 5 days every other day

    "Rule of 7's"
        • check estradiol 7 days after last pill (CD#16) to assess recruitment
        • check progesterone 7 days after estradiol to confirm ovulation
        • check ß-hCG 7 days after progesterone and perform pelvic exam/sono to assess prior
          to next clomiphene cycle

• increase clomiphene by 50 mg until ovulation obtained, 50% will ovulate on 50 mg
• follow follicular size with ultrasound
• consider IUI especially in couple with unexplained infertility
    • give 5,000-10,000 mIU hCG when follicle > 17 mm
    • ovulation will occur about 41 hr after hCG (Profasi)
• 15% of patients develop poor cervical mucus
• treatment usually limited to 4 ovulatory cycles as most pregnancies occur during 1st four cycles

Gonadotropins (FSH or FSH/LH combinations)
• candidates
    • hypothalamic-pituitary failure (Pergonal)
    • hypothalamic-pituitary dysfunction (Metrodin)
        • PCOS or other anovulatory menstrual disorders
    • unexplained infertility or minimal endometriosis
• informed consent essential
    • risk of multiple gestation (20%)
    • risk of ovarian hyperstimulation depends on stimulation
• administer hCG (Profasi) when estradiol 500-1500 pg/mL and lead follicle > 15 mm
    • give 12-36 h after last gonadotropin dose
    • timed intercourse that day and 2 days later or perform IUI

RECURRENT SPONTANEOUS ABORTION

Definition
• three or more consecutive spontaneous abortions
• primary: no previous pregnancy > 20 weeks with same partner
• secondary: three spontaneous abortions after pregnancy > 20 weeks

Fast Facts
• 10-15% of all pregnancies will not continue past first trimester
• risk of abortion is significantly greater with increasing maternal age (>40)

Etiologies
• genetic (autosomal trisomy, monosomy X)
• anatomic (uterine malformations, incompetent cervix, fibroids)
• endocrine (luteal phase defect, thyroid dysfunction, diabetes)
• infectious (bacteria, mycoplasma, viruses)
• immunologic (SLE, primary antiphospholipid syndrome)
• environmental (smoking, chemicals, radiation)

Diagnostic Test
• good history
• chromosomes (abortus, parents)
• HSG or hysteroscopy
• endocrine assessment (EMBx, TFT's, prolactin)
• cervical cultures
• immunologic profile (anticardiolipins etc.)

Treatment
• in many cases etiology remains a mystery so therapy is difficult
• immunotherapy with paternal leukocytes has been disappointing
• use of intravenous gamma globulin potentially helpful

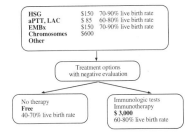

Courtesy of Dr. James R. Scott, University of Utah.

INFERTILITY

CLASSIFICATIONS OF MULLERIAN ANOMALIES

Class I. Dysgenesis of the Mullerian ducts
Class II. Disorders of vertical fusion of the Mullerian ducts
      A. transverse vaginal septum
          1. obstructed
          2. unobstructed
      B. cervical agenesis or dysgenesis
Class III. Disorders of lateral fusion of the Mullerian ducts
      A. asymmetric- obstructed disorder of uterus or vagina usually associated with ipsilateral renal agenesis
          1. Unicornuate uterus with noncommunicating rudimentary anlage or horn
          2. Unilateral obstruction of cavity of double uterus
          3. Unilateral vaginal obstruction associated with double uterus
      B. symmetric-unobstructed
          1. didelphic uterus
              a. complete longitudinal vaginal septum
              b. partial longitudinal vaginal septum
              c. no longitudinal vaginal septum
          2. septate uterus
              a. complete
                  (1) complete longitudinal vaginal septum
                  (2) partial longitudinal vaginal septum
                  (3) no longitudinal vaginal septum
              b. partial
                  (1) complete longitudinal vaginal septum
                  (2) partial longitudinal vaginal septum
                  (3) no longitudinal vaginal septum
          3. bicornuate uterus
              a. complete
                  (1) complete longitudinal vaginal septum
                  (2) partial longitudinal vaginal septum
                  (3) no longitudinal vaginal septum
              b. partial
                  (1) complete longitudinal vaginal septum
                  (2) partial longitudinal vaginal septum
                  (3) no longitudinal vaginal septum
          4. T-shaped uterine cavity (DES related)
          5. unicornuate uterus
              a. with rudimentary horn
                  (1) with endometrial cavity
                      (a) communicating
                      (b) noncommunicating
                  (2) without endometrial cavity
              b. without rudimentary horn
Class IV. Unusual configuration of vertical or lateral fusion defects

CLASSIFICATIONS OF MULLERIAN ANOMALIES

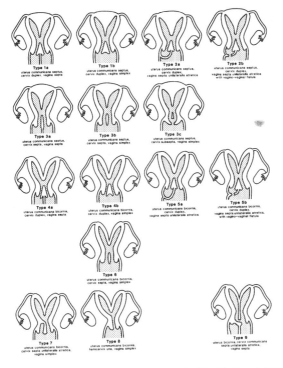

Source: Toaff ME, Lev TA, Toaff R. Communicating uteri: review and classification with introduction of two previously unreported types. *Fertil Steril.* 1984;41(5):661-79. Reproduced with the permission of the publisher, the American Society of Reproductive Medicine.

INFERTILITY

ASSISTED REPRODUCTIVE TECHNOLOGY

Fast Facts
- Louise Brown born July 25, 1978
- since 1985 > 50,000 deliveries worldwide

In vitro Fertilization - Embryo Transfer (IVF/ET)
- eggs are retrieved from ovaries and fertilized in Petri dish
- embryos reintroduced into uterus 2-6 days later
- indications
  - 52.2% tubal (mechanical) factor
  - 19% unexplained
  - 17.8% male factor
  - 1.7% endometriosis
  - 0.8% immunologic infertility (anti-sperm antibodies)
  - 8.5% other

Gamete Intrafallopian Transfer (GIFT)
- eggs/sperm mixed together following oocyte retrieval
- gametes then placed into distal fallopian tube by laparoscopy
- indications
  - healthy fallopian tubes
  - endometriosis (mild)
  - unexplained infertility
  - previous evidence of embryo formation during IVF or ZIFT

Zygote Intrafallopian Transfer (ZIFT)
- similar to IVF in all preliminary steps
- embryos transferred into fallopian tube by laparoscopy or trans-cervical route
- indications
  - same as IVF/ET but no tubal disease
- advantages
  - more physiologic
  - possible acquisition of tubal growth factors
- disadvantages
  - requires additional anesthesia (oocyte retrieval and laparoscopic embryo transfer)
    - ZIFT under local anesthesia has been reported

ASSISTED REPRODUCTIVE TECHNOLOGY

A.R.T.= Assisted Reproductive Technologies.

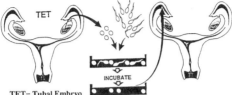

TET= Tubal Embryo
Transfer,(also termed ZIFT= Zygote Intra Fallopian Transfer)

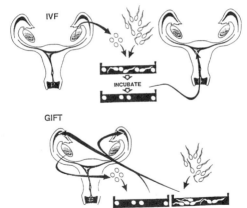

GIFT= Gamete Intra Fallopian Transfer

Courtesy of Dr. Ricardo Asch

INFERTILITY

COMPONENTS OF A TYPICAL ART CYCLE

Short (Flare) GnRH-a Protocol

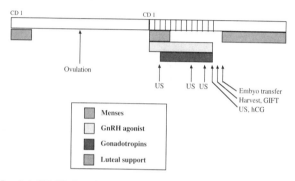

CD 1

CD 1

Ovulation

US

US US

Embyo transfer
Harvest, GIFT
US, hCG

	Menses
	GnRH agonist
	Gonadotropins
	Luteal support

Long (Luteal) GnRH-a Protocol

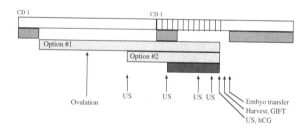

CD 1

CD 1

Option #1

Option #2

Ovulation

US

US

US US

Embyo transfer
Harvest, GIFT
US, hCG

INFERTILITY

STAGES IN FERTILIZATION

A. Follicular oocyte prior to the LH surge. The oocyte has an intact germinal vesicle (GV) and cumulus cell processes penetrate the zona pellucida (ZP) and form gap junctions with the oocyte.

B. Follicular oocyte soon after the LH surge (or hCG injection). Maturation changes are triggered in the oocyte and these include the synthesis of new proteins, breakdown of the GV and disruption of the cumulus-oocyte connections.

C. Follicular oocyte undergoing the final stages of maturation. The GV breakdown is complete and the oocyte is at metaphase of the first meiotic division. Cortical granules commence migration to the oocyte periphery. The cumulus cells begin elongation and mucification.

D. Preovulatory oocyte immediately after aspiration from the follicle. The oocyte has completed the first meiotic division and is at metaphase of the second meiotic division. The first polar body has been extruded, cortical granules are located just under the plasma membrane and the cumulus cells have dispersed in a mucin matrix.

E. Aspirated oocyte during 6 h in culture prior to insemination. Cortical granule migration and cytoplasmic maturation are completed.

F. Insemination of the oocyte with motile spermatozoa. Entry of the fertilizing sperm triggers cortical granule exocytosis and extrusion of the second polar body. Cortical granule release alters the AP and prevents further sperm penetration.

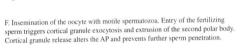

G. Fertilization in vitro. The oocyte has completed the second meiotic division and extruded the second polar body. The male and female pronuclei are forming.

H. Visualization of pronuclei 9-20 h after insemination.

I. Completion of the first cleavage division 24-35 h after insemination.

Source: Wood C, Trounson A. *Clinical in vitro fertilization.* Berlin New York: Springer-Verlag, 1984. Reproduced with the permission of the publisher.

263

INFERTILITY

1998 ASSISTED REPRODUCTIVE TECHNOLOGY SUCCESS RATES

Age	Cycles Initiated	% Retrieval	% Transfer	% Pregnancy	% Live Birth
Fresh non-donor eggs					
< 35 years	27,858	91	86	37	32
35-37	14,146	86	81	32	26
38-40	12,037	82	76	24	18
> 40	7,609	77	70	13	8

ART Success Rates for all Ages Combined

Fresh non-donor eggs	
Pregnancies/cycle initiated	30.5%
Live birth/cycle initiated	24.9%
Live birth/retrieval	28.9%
Live birth/transfer	30.8%

ART Outcomes for all Ages

Fresh non-donor eggs	
No pregnancy	68.9%
Single-fetus pregnancy	18.7%
Multiple-fetus pregnancy	11.8%
Ectopic pregnancy	0.6%

ART Pregnancy Outcomes for all Ages

Fresh non-donor eggs	
Singleton birth	50.9%
Multiple infant birth	30.9%
Miscarriage	16.1%
Induced abortion	1.6%
Stillbirth	0.5%

Source: *1998 Assisted Reproductive Technology Success Rates.* Centers for Disease Control and Prevention. U. S. Department of Health and Human Services.

1998 ASSISTED REPRODUCTIVE TECHNOLOGY SUCCESS RATES

Pregnancy and Live Birth Rates by Age (non-donor eggs)

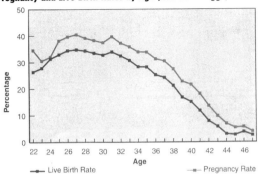

Live Births per Embryo Transfer by Age

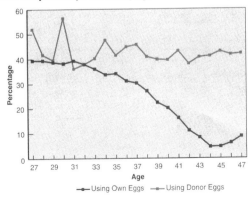

Source: *1998 Assisted Reproductive Technology Success Rates.* Centers for Disease Control and Prevention. U. S. Department of Health and Human Services.

INFERTILITY

OVARIAN HYPERSTIMULATION SYNDROME (OHSS)

Fast Facts
• OHSS is a self-limiting disease
• symptoms usually resolve in 1 week
• rarely occurs if hCG withheld
• more severe if pregnancy occurs

Classifications

	Adverse Reaction					
	Mild				Severe	
	1		2		3	
Laboratory and Clinical Findings	1	2	3	4	5	6
Excessive steroid production	+	+	+	+	+	+
Ovarian enlargement		+	+	+	+	+
Abdominal discomfort		+	+	+	+	+
Palpable ovarian cysts		?	+	+	+	+
Abdominal distention			+	+	+	+
Nausea			+	+	+	+
Vomiting				+	+	+
Diarrhea				?	+	+
Ascites					+	+
Hydrothorax						+
Severe hemoconcentration						+
Thromboembolic phenomena						?

Source: Lunenfeld B. et al. Short and long term survey of patients with hMG/hCG and follow-up of offspring. In: Genazani AR, Volpe A eds. *Proceedings of the 1st International Congress on Gynecologic Endocrinology*, 1987.

Medical Treatment
• maintain blood volume
• correct fluid/electrolyte balance (I/O's, daily weight)
• prevent thromboembolic events (plasma expanders)
• relieve secondary complications of ascites/hydrothorax

Surgical Treatment
• reserved for abdominal catastrophe
    • torsion, rupture, hemorrhage
• relieving pulmonary symptoms

Prevention
• "coasting" - stopping gonadotropins and awaiting drop in estradiol before giving hCG
• cancel cycle

MANAGEMENT OF OHSS

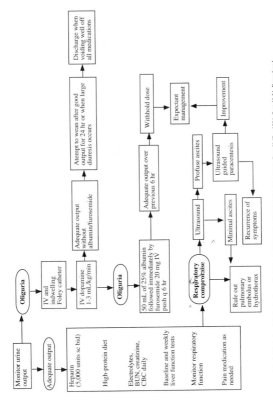

Source: Morris RS, Paulson RJ. Ovarian hyperstimulation syndrome: classification and management. *Cont ObGyn* 1994; Sept:43-54. Reproduced with permission.

267

INFERTILITY

MICROMANIPULATION IN ASSISTED REPRODUCTION
Fast Facts
- methods used to improve oocyte fertilization in vitro
- first human pregnancy following SuZI reported by Ng in 1988
- first live birth following SuZI reported in 1990 by Fishel
- 1,000 pregnancies worldwide
- severe male factor infertility not defined by 30% fertilization rate with ICSI even in cases of total motile count < 500,000
- fertilization and pregnancies have been obtained after microsurgical epididymal sperm aspiration (MESA) and IVF
- fertilization also reported after IVF-ICSI with testicular biopsy sperm

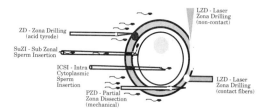

ZD - Zona Drilling (acid tyrode)

SuZI - Sub Zonal Sperm Insertion

ICSI - Intra Cytoplasmic Sperm Insertion

PZD - Partial Zona Dissection (mechanical)

LZD - Laser Zona Drilling (non-contact)

LZD - Laser Zona Drilling (contact fibers)

INFERTILITY

DES EXPOSURE
Fast Facts
• 90% of those with clear cell carcinoma have adenosis of vagina
• 20% have cervical hood, vaginal ridge, cockscomb cervix
• 63% have uterus with T-shaped cavity and constrictions at cornu
• 64% were fertile

Pregnancy Outcome (First Pregnancy)

Result	DES Exposed (N=150)	Unexposed (N=181)
Term	59 (52%)	106 (83%)
Preterm (>26 weeks or < 2500 g)	23 (20%)	8 (6%)
2nd Trimester loss (14-26 weeks)	5 (3%)	2 (1%)
1st Trimester loss (<13 weeks)	19 (13%)	12 (7%)
Ectopic	8 (7%)	0

Source: Herbst AL, Hubby MM, Azizi F, Makii MM. Reproductive and gynecologic surgical experience in diethylstilbestrol-exposed daughters. *Am J Obstet Gynecol* 1981;141(8):1019-28.

Exam
DES exposed female offspring
• start at 14 years or menarche or any age with symptoms

1. Inspect the introitus and hymen to assess vaginal patency
2. Palpate the vaginal membrane with the index finger note areas of induration or exophytic regions
3. Perform speculum exam with the largest speculum that can comfortably inserted. Adenosis will appear red and granular (strawberry surface.)
4. Obtain cytologic specimens from the cervical os and the upper 1/3 of the vagina
5. Perform colposcopic exam on initial visit
6. Biopsy indurated, exophytic lesions or colposcopically abnormal areas
7. Perform bimanual exam

Follow-up
• if no DES changes then yearly exam with Pap, colposcopy as indicated
• if has DES changes then q 6 month exams with Paps and colposcopy q 2 yr
• male DES changes:
    • epididymal cysts, undescended testes, low sperm counts but NO malignancy

269

LOCATION OF THE URETER

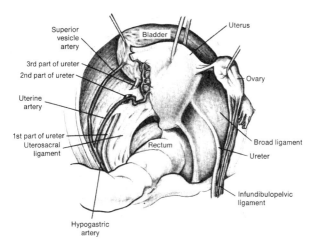

Source: DiSaia PJ, Creasman WT. Invasive cervical cancer. In: *Clinical Gynecologic Oncology*. 4th ed. St. Louis: Mosby Year Book, 1993. Reproduced with the permission of the publisher.

ANATOMY

PELVIC BLOOD SUPPLY

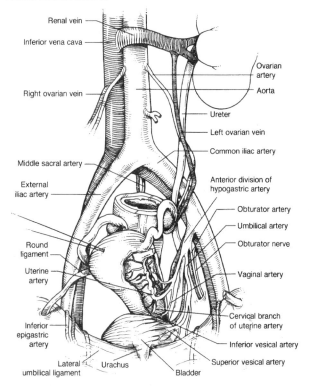

Source: DiSaia PJ. Clinical anatomy of the female pelvis. In: Scott JR, DiSaia PJ, Hammond CB, Spellacy WN, ed. *Danforth's Obstetrics and Gynecology.* 7th ed. Philadelphia: Lippincott, 1994. Reproduced with the permission of the publisher.

FETAL CIRCULATION

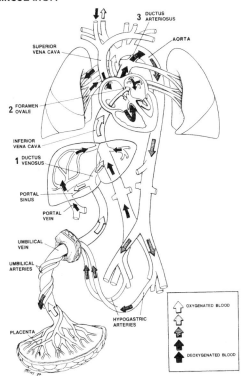

3 DUCTUS ARTERIOSUS

AORTA

SUPERIOR VENA CAVA

2 FORAMEN OVALE

INFERIOR VENA CAVA

1 DUCTUS VENOSUS

PORTAL SINUS

PORTAL VEIN

UMBILICAL VEIN

UMBILICAL ARTERIES

HYPOGASTRIC ARTERIES

PLACENTA

OXYGENATED BLOOD

DEOXYGENATED BLOOD

Source: Cunningham FG, MacDonald PC, Gant NF et al. The morphological and functional development of the fetus. In: *Williams Obstetrics.* 20th ed. Stamford, Conn.: Appleton & Lange, 1997. Reproduced with the permission of the publisher.

ANATOMY

BONY PELVIS

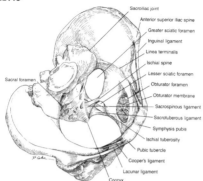

Sacroiliac joint
Anterior superior iliac spine
Greater sciatic foramen
Inguinal ligament
Linea terminalis
Ischial spine
Lesser sciatic foramen
Obturator foramen
Obturator membrane
Sacrospinous ligament
Sacrotuberous ligament
Symphysis pubis
Ischial tuberosity
Pubic tubercle
Cooper's ligament
Lacunar ligament
Coccyx

Sacral foramen

LUMBAR/SACRAL NERVE PLEXUSES

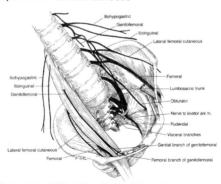

Iliohypogastric
Genitofemoral
Ilioinguinal
Lateral femoral cutaneous

Iliohypogastric
Ilioinguinal
Genitofemoral

Femoral
Lumbosacral trunk
Obturator
Nerve to levator ani m.
Pudendal
Visceral branches
Genital branch of genitofemoral

Lateral femoral cutaneous
Femoral
Femoral branch of genitofemoral

From Burnett LS. Anatomy. In: Jones HW, Wentz AC, Burnett LS. ed. *Novak's Textbook of Gynecology.* 11th ed. Baltimore: Williams & Wilkins, 1988. Reproduced with the permission of the publisher.

JOEL-COHEN INCISION FOR LAPAROTOMY

Position of the incision being made. The skin incision is not curved, but made straight from one indentation to the other 4 cm below the anterior superior iliac spine. Cutting through the subcutaneous tissue (superficial) and down to and through the fascia in the midline for 2.5-4 cm.

Cutting fascia under subcutaneous tissue.   Stretching cranio-caudally between muscles.

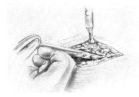
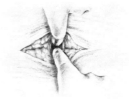

Rectus muscle being pulled apart by operator and assistant. The peritoneum is held by two forceps (cranially and caudally in the midline, be sure that no bowel is caught) and incise transversely. Stretch sideways to the size of the skin and fascial opening.

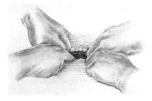

Source: Joel-Cohen S. *Abdominal and Vaginal Hysterectomy: new techniques based on time and motion studies.* (2nd ed). Philadelphia: J.B. Lippincott, 1977. Reproduced with permission of the publisher.

STANFORD UNIVERSITY HOPITAL CLINICAL MICROBIOLOGY LABORATORY

Antibiotic Susceptibility of Bacterial Isolates

GRAM NEGATIVE — Percent Susceptible by Disk Diffusion Assay (b)	Lactose Fermentation on Primary Selective Media (g)	No. Tested (a)	PENICILLINS			CEPHALOSPORINS					
			Ampicillin	Piperacillin (dd)	Ticarcillin/ clavulanate	Cefazolin	Cefotetan	Cefuroxime I.V.	Cefuroxime P.O.	Cefotaxime	Ceftazidime (dd)
Acinetobacter anitratum	NF	72		25	85						90
Acinetobacter lwoffi	NF	21		90	95						93
Aeromonas species	LF	16	0	81	81	50				94	100
Alcaligenes faecalis (b)	NF	12		67	67						67
Alcaligenes xylosoxidans (b)	NF	8		100	100						88
Citrobacter diversus	NLF	23	91	91	100	100	100	96	29	100	100
Citrobacter freundii	LF	93	46	46	53	10	58	52	35	54	55
Enterobacter aerogenes	LF/NLF	125	49	67	47	5	45	46	21	52	55
Enterobacter cloacae	LF/NLF	267	67	68	62	3	47	53	7	67	71
Escherichia coli	LF	1356	63	68	86	92	100	97	68	99(h)	100(h)
Hafnia alvei	NLF	20	25	25	80	100	100	70	21	75	75
Klebsiella oxytoca	LF	100	0	84	93	63	100	93	74	98(h)	98(h)
Klebsiella pneumoniae	LF	380	0	76	92	96	100	92	54	100(h)	100(h)
Morganella morganii	NLF	26	0	96	100	0	100	19	9	96	100
Proteus mirabilis	NLF	177	89	94	99	95	100	99	95	100	100
Proteus vulgaris	NLF	15	20	100	100	13	100	33	31	100	100
Providencia species	NLF	14	57	100	100	79	100	100	100	100	100
Pseudomonas aeruginosa (dd)	NF	726		84	73			2	0		87
Burkholderia (Pseudo.) cepacia (b)	NF	3		33	0						33
Pseudomonas fluorescens grp. (b)	NF	7		86	14						86
Salmonella species	NLF	15	67							100	
Serratia marcescens	NLF	114	0	97	97		96			97	99
Shigella species	NLF	30	57							100	
Xanthomonas maltophilia (b)	NF	96		21	75						57
Haemophilus influenzae (bb)	NLF	142	67(f) (Amoxicillin/clavulanate 100%)				(Rifampin 82%)	100	99	100 (Sulfisoxazole 73%)	
Neisseria meningitidis	NF	11	100 (Penicillin)							100	
Moraxella catarrhalis	NF	26	4(f) (Amoxicillin/clavulanate 100%)							100 (Erythromycin 100%)	
Cost (Antibiotic only) — Injectable			$0.43 gm	11.00 gm 4 gm	10.53 3.1 gm	1.91 1 gm	8.75 gm	5.03 750 mg		6.96 gm	10.64 gm
Cost (Antibiotic only) — Oral			$0.09 500 mg						4.77 500 mg		

STANFORD UNIVERSITY HOPITAL CLINICAL MICROBIOLOGY LABORATORY (CONT.)

	LACTAMS		AMINOGLYCOSIDES (I.C.e.)			OTHER		URINE ONLY (I.C.e.)			
	Aztreonam (cc)	Imipenem	Gentamicin	Tobramycin	Amikacin	Ciprofloxacin	Trimeth./sulfa	1st genera-tion Cephalo-sporins (oral)	Nitro-furantion	Sulfisoxa-zole	Tetra-cycline
	1	100	88	96	96	88	90				38
	29	100	100	95	100	90	95				80
	100	100	100	100	100	100	69				
	0	100	42	42	58	50	50				
		88	0	0	0	0	88				
	100	100	100	100	100	100	100	d	d	d	d
	56	99	99	99	98	98	78	3	97	74	74
	54	99	99	99	99	91	96	6	39	78	78
	70	99	99	97	99	97	94	2	58	78	46
	99	100	98	98	99	99	82	66	97	69	72
	100	100	100	100	100	100	100	75	92	79	88
	96	100	98	97	99	97	94	59	59	76	63
	100	100	100	100	100	100	92	d	d	d	d
	100	99	94	100	100	99	92	95	d	85	d
	100	100	100	100	100	99	95	d	d	d	d
	100	100	60	36	100	100	100	d	d	d	d
	68	85	81	96	33	83	64	0	0		
	0	33	33	33	33	86	14				
	14	86	86	100	98	86	87				
						92	43			75	
	99	100	99	96	98	26	99	(Chloramphenicol 100%)	0		0
	8	3	22	25	27	100	90		9		9
Cost	11.48 gm	18.66 500 mg	0.83 80 mg	3.52 80 mg	32.26 500 mg	24.00 400 mg / 2.52 500 mg	1.00 amp / 1.00 / 0.08 DS tabs	0.20 500 mg	0.45 50 mg	0.03 500 mg	0.03 250 mg

Footnotes on page 281-282.

STANFORD UNIVERSITY HOPITAL CLINICAL MICROBIOLOGY LABORATORY (CONT.)

GRAM POSITIVE — Percent Susceptible by Disk Diffusion Assay	No. Tested (a)	Penicillin (j,l) %	Ampicillin (L,m,n) %	Nafcillin, Oxacillin (k), Methicillin %	1st generation Cephalosporin (k) %	Vancomycin %	Erythromycin (g) %S	Erythromycin %I	Clindamycin (q) %S	Clindamycin %I	Chloramphenicol %	Gentamicin %	% with High Level Aminoglycoside Resistance (m,n) — Gentamicin	Streptomycin	Trimeth./sulfa.	Rifampin	Ciprofloxacin	Tetracycline (c,e)	Nitrofurantoin (c,e)
Staphylococci																			
Staphylococcus aureus (AB) (v)	1102	11		97	97	100	72	14	91			93			96	99	87	83	
MRSA (only) (k)	37	0		0	0	100	16	35				48			81	30	97		
Staph. coagulase negative	1099	18		22	47	100	40	13	66			57			63	48	57	57	
Staph. epidermidis		15		20	47	100	35		57			63			49	83	100		
Staph. haemolyticus	13	31		31	31	100	33	42	92			29			92	92	83		
Staph. hominis	19	62		60	60	100	53	73	100			94			94	95	100		
Staph. saprophyticus	26	72		72	72	100						100			92	100	75	120
Streptococci																			
Grp. A (Strep. pyogenes)	50	100			100	100	84		74	22									
Grp. B (Strep. agalactiae)	266	100			100	100	82	13	79	17	89								
Grp. C	11	100			100	100	67	25	58	16									
Grp. F	18	100			100	100	89	6	89	6									
Grp. G	23	100			100	100	78	22	70	26									
Grp. D enterococci	817	>99	77			100													
Enterococcus faecalis	100		>99			100							12	17			33	21	96
Enterococcus faecium	42		6										15	23			62	23	100
Grp. D non-enterococci	13		77			100							9	79			0	100	57
Viridans (s)	83		81			100													
Strep. pneumoniae (p)	103		83			100						92						75	
Listeria monocytogenes	4	100	100									100			100				

Cost (Antibiotic only):

	Penicillin	Ampicillin	Nafcillin / Dicloxacillin	Cefazolin / Cefaclor	Vancomycin	Erythromycin	Clindamycin	Chloramphenicol	Gentamicin	Trimeth./sulfa.	Ciprofloxacin	Tetracycline / Doxy	Nitrofurantoin
Inpatient (Amt./$)	Pen G 1.00	Amp. $0.43	1.00	Cefazolin 1.94	6.92	1.94	2.05	1.50	0.83	0.67	24.00		
Inpatient dose	500 mg	gm		gm	gm	500 mg	600 mg	gm	80 mg	300 mg	400 mg		
Oral (Amt./$)	0.06	0.05	Diclox. 0.16	0.20		0.05	0.89				2.52	0.03 / 1.15	0.45
Oral dose	250 mg	gm	500 mg	Cefaclor 500 mg		250 mg	150 mg				500 mg	250 mg / 100 mg	50 mg

Footnotes on page 281–282.

STANFORD UNIVERSITY HOPITAL CLINICAL MICROBIOLOGY LABORATORY (CONT.)

ANAEROBES — Percent Susceptible by MIC (Micro-broth dilution) (t,aa)

	No. Tested (aa)	Penicillin	Piperacillin	Ticarcillin/ clavulanate	Imipenem	Cefotetan	Chlorampheni- col	Clindamycin	Metronidazole
Bacteroides fragilis	29	0	79	97	100	86	100	90	100
Bacteroides fragilis group (u)	30	0	73	100	100	35	93	83	100
Bacteroides species, other (v)	30	27	100	100	100	100	100	97	97
Clostridium perfringens	15	100	100	100	100	100	100	100	100
Clostridium species	16	94	100	100	100	69	100	69	94
Fusobacterium species	9	89	100	100	100	100	100	89	100
Peptostreptococcus species (w)	8	100	100	100	100	100	100	100	88
Propionibacterium acnes	5	100	100	100	100	100	100	100	0

MYCOBACTERIUM	No. Tested	Isoniazid 0.1mcg/ml	Isoniazid 2.0mcg/ml	Strepto- myocin 4.0mcg/ml	Strepto- myocin 10.0mcg/ml	Rifampin 0.5mcg/ml	Ethambutol 4.0mcg/ml
M. tuberculosis (x)	12	83	83	100	100	100	100

INTERPRETIVE CRITERIA FOR PENICILLIN AND AMPICILLIN FOR DIFFERENT ORGANISMS MINIMUM INHIBITORY CONCENTRATION (ug/ml)

Organisms	Enterics	Staphylococci M. catarrhalis	Enterococci	S. pneumoniae N. gonorrhoeae(s)	Other Streptococci	Listeria	Haemophilus
Antibiotic	Amp.	Pen./Amp.	Pen./Amp.	Pen.	Pen./Amp.	Amp.	Amp.
Interpretation Susceptible (S) or Very Susceptible (VS)	≤ 8	< 0.12/0.25	≤ 8	< 0.06	< 0.12	< 2.0	≤ 1.0
Intermediate (I)	16	> 0.25/0.5	16	0.12-1.0	0.25-2.0		2.0
Resistant (R)	> 32		> 16	> 2.0	> 4.0	> 4.0	> 4.0

Acknowledgement John DeBell for compilation of susceptibility data.

Footnotes on page 281-282.

MICROBIOLOGY

Footnotes

a. Duplicate isolates with identical susceptibility from the same source excluded.

b. MIC's determined by micro-broth dilution for the species indicated, and currently for gram negative rods recovered from blood or CSF.

c. Not all isolates tested with these antibiotics.

d. Less than 10 isolates tested.

e. Tested for urinary tract isolates only.

f. All resistant isolates were beta-lactamase positive.

g. On preliminary reports, gram negative rods may be characterized as lactose fermenters (LF), or non-lactose fermenters (NLF). Some nonlactose fermenters may be further characterized as non-fermenters (NF). LF includes: *E. coli, Klebsiellas,* most *Citrobacter,* most *Enterobacter.* NLF includes: *Proteus, Providencia, Serratia, Salmonella, Shigella,* and some *Citrobacter* and *Enterobacter.* NF includes: *Pseudomonas, Acinetobacter, Alcaligenes, Xanthomonas,* which intrinsically are resistant to many antibiotics.

h. Isolates of *E. coli* and *Klebsiella* species which are resistant to either ceftazidime or cefotaxime usually produce extended spectrum beta-lactamases and, despite reports of in vitro susceptibility to some cephalosporins, should not be treated with this group of antibiotics because of reported treatment failures.

i. Viridans (alpha hemolytic) streptococci include species: *Streptococcus anginosus S. mitis S. mutans S. sanguis* and *S. salivarius.*

j. Penicillin resistant staphylococci should be considered resistant to all penicillinase sensitive penicillins including ampicillin, amoxicillin, mezlocillin, piperacillin, and ticarcillin.

k. Methicillin resistant staphylococci (MRSA) should be considered resistant to all cephalosporins, imipenem and beta-lactams including combinations with clavulanate, sulbactam, or tazobactam. For staphylococci, streptococci, and other penicillin susceptible organisms, "Susceptible" results should be regarded as very susceptible (see Interpretation of Results and footnote m).

m. Most enterococci (i.e. *E. faecalis*) will be reported as susceptible to ampicillin and penicillins, as well as vancomycin, piperacillin, and betalactamase inhibitor combinations which exhibit activity similar to penicillin and ampicillin however; high dose penicillin or ampicillin is recommended for treatment of serious invasive tissue infections such as endocarditis which also may require combination therapy with an aminoglycosides. Ampicillin alone may be used to treat enterococcal urinary tract infection. Vancomycin should be reserved for serious infections in patients with significant penicillin allergy.

n. Synergistic bactericidal action with penicillin or ampicillin and an aminoglycoside does not occur for strains of enterococci demonstrating high level resistance (gentamicin MIC >500 mcg/ml or streptomycin MIC >2000 mcg/ml) to the particular aminoglycoside. For isolates of enterococci which demonstrate high level resistance to gentamicin, synergistic killing will not be obtained with a betalactam and other aminoglycosides including tobramycin, amikacin, or kanamycin.

o. A pneumococcal isolate that is susceptible to penicillin (MIC 2 mcg/ml) can be considered susceptible to other beta-lactams which may be used for approved indications. Infectious diseases consultation is recommended when *S. pneumoniae* causing serious infections are either penicillin resistant (MIC 2 mcg/ml) or classified as intermediate (MIC 0.5-1 ug/ml) or resistant (MIC 2 mcg/ml) to cefotaxime/ceftriaxone. Meningitis due to isolates which are reported as intermediate (I) to penicillin (MIC 0.12-1.0 mcg/ml) or penicillin resistant should be treated with alternative antibiotics due to reported treatment failure with penicillin. Resistance to cephalosporins is frequently increased in pneumococcal isolates which are intermediate or resistant to penicillin, and beta-lactam inhibitors such as clavulanate or sulbactam do not improve beta-lactam activity. *S. pneumoniae* which are resistant to ceftriaxone/cefotaxime (MIC 2 mcg/ml) have been associated with treatment failure in cases of meningitis treated with these antibiotics and also should be considered resistant to oral cephalosporins. For isolates of *S. pneumoniae* reported as intermediate to cefotaxime/ ceftriaxone (MIC 0.5-1 mcg/ml), recommendations for optimum treatment of meningitis or clinical efficacy of oral cephalosporins for treatment of localized infections remains to be established.

p. Usual range of ampicillin MIC's for group B streptococci is 0.06-0.25 mcg/ml. Although isolates with MIC's >0.1 mcg/ml are classified as intermediate, ampicillin or penicillin remains the antibiotic of choice. (See table Interpretation of Results).

q. % Susceptible (S)/% Intermediate (I). Gram positive isolates which have MIC's of 1-4 mcg/ml to erythromycin. or 1-2 mcg/ml to clindamycin are classified as I, indicating that adequate levels of drug will not be obtained using some oral preparations and doses, and that IV therapy may be needed. True resistance to erythromycin remains uncommon in *S. Peogenes* and *S. pneumoniae* (only 2% and 6% of *S. aureus* were classified as I to clindamycin and erythromycin respectively).

r. Listeria should be considered resistant to cephalosporins.

s. Susceptibility testing of gonococci has been discontinued.

t. Anaerobic susceptibility results correlate poorly with clinical response and therefore are of limited value in management of most cases. Current guidelines recommend that for purposes of management, anaerobic susceptibility testing be limited to situations such as treatment failure, brain abscess, endocarditis, osteomyelitis, joint infections, infections of prosthetic devices or vascular grafts, and refractory or recurrent bacteremia. A very high proportion of anaerobes are susceptible to metronidazole, chloramphenicol, ticarcillin clavulanate, and imipenem. Cefotetan and clindamycin have generally been very effective agents, although clinically significant resistance may occur. Also see footnote (dd).

u. Bacteroides fragilis group includes *B. distasonis, B. ovatus, B. thetaiotaomicron, B vulgaris, B. uniformis,* and *B. caccae. B. fragilis* is separated from other members of this group for purposes of this report.

v. Most of the organisms in this group have been reclassified as Prevotella and Porphyromonas.
w. Due to low numbers of isolates recovered, data for a three year period is presented.
x. Two isolates of *M. tuberculosis*, which were resistant to isoniazid, were susceptible to the secondary drugs ethionamide, cycloserine, and kanamycin.

RECOMMENDATIONS BY ANTIBIOTIC UTILIZATION TEAM

y. For *S. aureus*, nafcillin and first generation cephalosporins are recommended drugs of choice at SUH due to low (3%) incidence of resistance to methicillin/nafcillin. Vancomycin should be reserved for infections due to suspected or documented methicillin/nafcillin resistant staphylococci.

z. Gentamicin is the recommended aminoglycoside for the treatment of aerobic gram negative infections. Tobramycin should be reserved for infection due to *P. aeruginosa*.

aa. Based on low percentage of resistance and cost advantages, metronidazole is the recommended drug of choice for *B. fragilis* infections.

bb. For infections with beta-lactamase producing *H. influenzae*, cefuroxime, cefotaxime, trimethoprim/sulfamethoxazole, or amoxicillin/ clavulanate are recommended options. Cefotaxime is recommended for CNS infections.

cc. Aztreonam should NOT be considered as a replacement for aminoglycosides in most situations. Aminoglycosides have superior in-vitro activity against aerobic gram negative organisms when compared to aztreonam. Unlike aztreonam, aminoglycosides have synergistic activity with other beta-lactams (piperacillin/penicillin) against aerobic gram negative organisms and enterococcus. Aztreonam should only be used for documented infection due to susceptible organisms in patients with anaphylactic reactions with a beta-lactam. In patients with renal insufficiency aminoglycosides can be administered safely when doses are adjusted for patient's renal function

dd. Ceftazidime and piperacillin are potent anti-pseudomonal agents available on the SUH formulary with similar activity against *Pseudomonas aeruginosa* (87% and 84% respectively). At SUH, ceftazidime is used more far more frequently than piperacillin for the treatment of aerobic gram negative infections. A recent study indicated that treatment of Enterobacter bacteremia with a third generation cephalosporin, such as ceftazidime, was associated with development of resistance during therapy. Patients who developed these resistant organisms were associated with increased mortality. This emergence of resistance was not observed with the use of piperacillin. Based on this data, use of piperacillin and an aminoglycoside is recommended for treatment of infections due to susceptible strains of *Enterobacter* species and *Pseudomonas aeruginosa*.

ANTIBIOTICS TESTED

Susceptibility information is provided for antibiotics on the SUMC formulary. Organism - antibiotic combinations routinely tested and reported are restricted to those recommended by the National Committee for Clinical Laboratory Standards (NCCLS) and have been reviewed by representatives from Infectious Diseases, Pharmacy and the Clinical Microbiology Laboratory. Antibiotics available on the formulary are active against > 95% of pathogens isolated at this institution.

INTERPRETATION OF SUSCEPTIBILITY RESULTS (NCCLS M2-A5 AND M7-A3)

Susceptible (S)—This categorization implies that an infection due to the strain tested may be appropriately treated with the dosage of antimicrobial agents recommended for that type of infection and infecting species, unless otherwise contraindicated.

Intermediate (I)—MIC' S for these isolates approach usually attainable blood and tissue levels and response rates may be lower than for susceptible isolates. The "intermediate" category implies clinical applicability in body sites where the drugs are physiologically concentrated (e.g. quinolones and beta-lactams in urine or when high dosage of drug can be used (e .g., beta-lactams)). The "intermediate" category also indicates a "buffer zone" which should prevent small uncontrolled technical factors from causing major discrepancies in interpretation, especially for drugs with narrow pharmacotoxicity margins.

Resistant (R)—Resistant strains are not inhibited by the usually achievable systemic concentrations of the agent with normal dosage schedules and/or fall in the range where specific microbial resistance mechanisms are likely (e.g., beta lactamases), and clinical efficacy has not been reliable in treatment studies. For penicillin and ampicillin interpretive categories and minimum inhibitory concentrations (MIC) correlates vary depending on the species. For some organisms these antibiotics may be the treatment of choice even when the isolate is reported to be "Intermediate " See footnotes l, m, o, p.

From the Clinical Microbiology Laboratory, Stanford University Hospital.

Lucy S. Tompkins, M.D., Ph.D., Director
Patricia A. Mickelsen, Ph.D., Co-Director
Susan D. Munro, M.T. (ASCP), Coordinator, Antibiotic Section

EPIDEMIOLOGY

DEFINITION
• the study of health and health problems in populations

Alternative Definitions
• medical student: The worst taught class in medical school
• resident: A very scary field in medicine filled with math
• David Grimes' Mother: A dermatology subspecialty (see Epidermatologist)

Epidemiologic Study Designs
• Descriptive Studies
• Analytic Studies
• Cohort Studies
• Case-control Studies
• Experimental Studies
• Randomized Clinical Trials

Basic Terms

Prevalence $\dfrac{\text{\# of people who have a disease at one point in time}}{\text{\# of persons at risk at that point}}$

Incidence $\dfrac{\text{\# of new cases of disease over a period of time}}{\text{\# of persons at risk during that period}}$

Sensitivity The proportion of subjects with the disease who have a positive test (a/a+c)

Specificity The proportion of subjects without the disease who have a negative test (d/b+d)

Predictive value • positive - likelihood a positive test indicates disease (a/a+b)
• negative - likelihood a negative test indicates lack of disease (d/d+c)

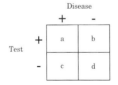

EPIDEMIOLOGY

DESCRIPTIVE STUDIES
Advantages
• data are relatively easy to obtain
• cost of obtaining data is relatively low
• ethical problems are minimal since the researcher does not decide which health services are to be received

Disadvantages
• no comparison group
• cause and effect relationships are suggested only

Study Design

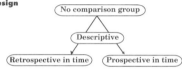

Analysis
• tables
• histogram
• line graphs
• scatter diagrams
• other graphic representation

ANALYTIC STUDIES
Essential Features
There are at least 2 study groups:
• a group of subjects with the outcome or exposure of interest and a group of individuals without the health
    problem or exposure of interest
• association between exposure and outcome can be examined
• study subtypes named according to the determination of the study groups

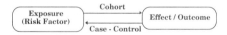

EPIDEMIOLOGY

COHORT STUDIES
Advantages
- avoids having to withhold treatment from those who wish to receive it
- uses prospective data collection allowing standardization of eligibility criteria, the maneuver and outcome assessment
- uses concurrent control group; co-intervention less likely to influence results since it should affect both groups
- uses prospective data collection
- can match for potential confounders during sample selection

Disadvantages
- impossible to ensure known confounding variables are equally distributed between groups
- impossible to ensure that some factor unidentified by the investigator is not responsible both for exposure to the maneuver and good outcomes
- difficult to achieve blindness to intervention with resulting bias likely (i.e. increased attention to experimental group)
- difficult to obtain concurrent controls if therapy is in vogue
- expensive in time, money, and subjects to do well

Study Design

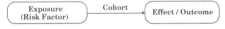

- at least two groups of subjects are studied
- entry into these groups is not randomized
- both groups of subjects are followed for a period of time to determine the frequency of the outcome in each group
- the risk of developing the outcome for those exposed and those not exposed will be compared to see if there is a difference
- to determine whether an association exists between an exposure (risk factor) and a future outcome (health problem)

Analysis

	Outcome		
	Yes	No	
Exposure Yes	a	b	N_1
Exposure No	c	d	N_0

$$\text{Relative Risk} = \frac{a/N_1}{c/N_0}$$

$$\text{Attributable Risk} = a/N_1 - c/N_0$$

EPIDEMIOLOGY

CASE CONTROL STUDIES

Advantages
- useful for health problems that occur infrequently
- useful for studying health problems with long latent interval
- less time-consuming and less expensive than cohort studies because of the convenient sampling strategy and relatively short study period

Disadvantages
- selection bias - cases and controls are selected from two separate populations
    - difficult to ensure that they are comparable with respect to extraneous risk factors and other sources of distortion
- information bias - exposure data is collected from records or by recall after disease occurrence
    - records may be incomplete and recall of past events is subject to human error and selective recall
- inappropriate for determining incidence rates
- inappropriate for determining the other possible health effects of an exposure

Study Design

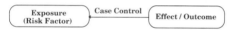

- two groups of subjects studied: one group that experiences the outcome (cases) and the other that does not (controls)
- entry into these two groups not influenced by the investigator and therefore cannot be randomized
- cases are identified during a given period of time
- the exposure of the two groups to specific risk factors in the past is investigated.
- the likelihood that the cases were exposed to specific risk factors is then compared to the likelihood that controls were exposed to the same risk factors to see if there is a significant difference

Analysis

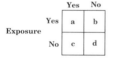

$$\text{Odds Ratio} = \frac{a/b}{c/d} = \frac{ad}{bc}$$

- proportion that cases and controls represent in the population is unknown
- estimate of the relative risk can be obtained by cross-product ratio
- odds ratio approximates relative risk if incidence of outcome is < 5%

RANDOMIZED CLINICAL TRIALS

Advantages

• controls selection bias effectively
• balances potential confounding variables
• allows standardization of eligibility criteria, exposures and outcome assessments
• statistically efficient because equal numbers of exposed and unexposed can be studied
• statistically efficient because statistical power is not lost when confounding is controlled for in the analysis
• theoretically attractive since many statistical methods are based on random assignment
• concurrent comparison groups

Disadvantages

• design and implementation of an RCT may be complex
• extrapolation to the general population may be limited by careful selection criteria employed to conduct RCT
• open to ethical challenges: can exposure be ethically withheld from one group

Study Design

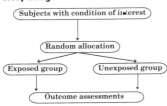

• two groups of subjects are studied, those exposed to each of two treatments
• subjects are randomly assigned to one of the two treatment groups
• subjects are analyzed as part of the group to which they were randomized even if they fail to complete therapy (not intuitively obvious)

Analysis

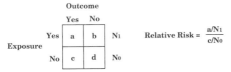

• essentially same analysis as for cohort study with determination of RR

EPIDEMIOLOGY

STUDY SIZE AND POWER ANALYSIS
Type I Error (alpha error)
Probability of a study showing a statistically significant difference when no real difference exists (null hypothesis true). A P-value of 0.05 indicates a 5% probability of obtaining a difference when there is none.

Type II Error (beta error)
False-negative result is the probability of failing to show a statistically significant difference when a true difference exists.

Power
The probability of a study detecting a statistically significant difference when a real difference exists. Complement to Type II error as Power = 1 - beta

BIAS
Selection Bias
The persons in one study group are different on some factor other than presence or absence of disease (case-control) or exposure (cohort) that was not measured and therefore, cannot be controlled for in the analysis.

Ascertainment Bias
The information regarding outcome in a cohort study or history of exposure in a case control study has not been obtained in an equal fashion for both subjects and controls.

Confounding
The two comparison groups differ in some characteristic which is self-associated with both the outcome and exposure being studied but not directly involved in the causal pathway.

Random Bias
The two comparison groups differ because of chance. Confidence intervals can be computed for the RR estimate thus allowing testing of the null hypothesis.

Special thanks to David Grimes, Ken Schulz, and the Berlex Foundation.

BASIC SPANISH

Numbers

one	uno (una)	sixteen	dieciséis
two	dos	seventeen	diecisiete
three	tres	eighteen	dieciocho
four	cuatro	nineteen	diecinueve
five	cinco	twenty	veinte
six	seis	thirty	trienta
seven	siete	forty	cuarenta
eight	ocho	fifty	cincuenta
nine	nueve	sixty	sesenta
ten	diez	seventy	setenta
eleven	once	eighty	ochenta
twelve	doce	ninety	noventa
thirteen	trece	hundred	cien
fourteen	catorce	thousand	mil
fifteen	quince		

Years

1930	mil novecientos treinta
1943	mil novecientos cuarenta y tres
1960	mil novecientos sesenta
1970	mil novecientos setenta
1974	mil novecientos setenta y cuatro

Days of the week

Monday	lunes
Tuesday	martes
Wednesday	miércoles
Thursday	jueves
Friday	viernes
Saturday	sábado
Sunday	domingo

Times

morning	la mañana
afternoon	la tarde
evening	la tarde
night	la noche
today	hoy
tomorrow	mañana
last night	anoche
yesterday	ayer
day before yesterday	anteayer

Months

January	enero
February	febrero
March	marzo
April	abril
May	mayo
June	junio
July	julio
August	agosto
September	septiembre
October	octubre
November	noviembre
December	diciembre

SPANISH PRIMER

Introductions

Good morning
Buenos días

How do you feel?
Cómo se siente? Cómo esta?

My name is ••••
Me llamo ••••

Please
Por favor

Obstetrical and Gynecologic History

At what age did you begin to menstruate?
A qué edad empezó su menstruación?

What was the first day of your last period?
Cuándo fue el primer día de su última regla? (menstruación, período)

When did you have your last period?
Cuándo fue su última regla?

Did you have a normal period?
Tuvo una regla normal? (Fue esta regla normal?)

Pregnancy
Embarazo, encinta, "gorda"

How many pregnancies have you had?
Cuántos embarazos ha tenido usted?

How many children have you had?
Cuántos niños ha tenido usted?

Are they all living?
Estan vivos todos?

What was the cause of death? At what age?
Cuál fue la causa de la muerte? A qué edad?

Have you had any problems with past pregnancies?
Ha tenido algunos problemas con sus embarazos pasados?

Bleeding? Hypertension? Toxemia?
Sangrando (hemorragia)? Alta presión de la sangre? Toxemia?

Have you had any problems with past deliveries?
Ha tenido problemas con sus partos pasados?

What was the duration of your longest (shortest) labor?
Cuántas horas duró su parto más largo (más corto)?

What was the date of your last pregnancy?
Cuál fue la fecha de su último embarazo?

What was the weight of your largest (smallest) baby at birth?
Cuánto pesó el bebé más grande (más pequeño) al nacer?

Were all your pregnancies term?
Fueron de tiempo (de nueve meses) sus otros niños?

Were there any problems with the children after birth?
Después de nacer, tuvo algún o algunos problemas con los niños?

Have you ever had a miscarriage? Was it the first, second? What date?
Ha tenido un malparto, aborto? Fue el primero, el segundo? Qué fecha?

Have you ever had a stillborn?
Ha tenido un niño que ha nacido muerto?

Have you ever had a cesarean section? What date?
Ha tenido usted una operación cesárea? Qué fecha?

Past Medical and Surgical History
Have you had any operations? For what? When? In which hospital?
Ha tenido algunas operaciones? Para qué? Cuándo? En cuál hospital?

Have you had any major illnesses?
Ha tenido algunas enfermedades graves?

Have you had any accidents, fractures?
Ha tenido algunos accidentes, fracturas?

Have you ever had a blood transfusion?
Ha tenido una transfusión (infusión) de sangre?

Have you been taking any medications?
Qué medicinas ha estado tomando?

Are you allergic to medicines or foods?
Es usted alérgica a medicinas o comidas?

Do you smoke? How many packs in a day (week)? Cigarettes
Fuma usted? Cuántos paquetes en un día (una semana)? Cigarillos

SPANISH PRIMER

Family History

Have you or anyone in your family had:
Usted o alguien en su familia ha tenido:

asthma	asma
cancer	cáncer
convulsions	convulsiones
diabetes	diabetes
epilepsy	epilepsia
gonorrhea	gonorrea
syphilis	sífilis
hay fever	fiebre del heno
heart disease	mala (enfermedad) del corazón
hepatitis (liver)	hepatitis (hígado)
hypertension	alta presión de la sangre
influenza	influenza, gripe
jaundice (yellow skin)	ictericia (la piel amarilla)
measles	sarampión
chicken pox	viruela
pneumonia	pulmonía, neumonía
rheumatic fever	fiebre reumática
scarlet fever	fiebre escarlatina
stroke	hemoragia cerebral
thyroid	tiroides
tuberculosis	tuberculosis
tumor	tumor
infections of the bladder, kidney	infecciones de la vejiga, de los riñones
infections of the chest, lungs	infecciones del pecho o de los pulmones

Anatomy

head	cabeza	**heart**	corazón
eyes	ojos	**lungs (lung)**	pulmones (pulmón)
ears	oídos	**abdomen**	abdomen (vientre)
nose	nariz	**liver**	hígado
mouth	boca	**intestines**	intestinos
tongue	lengua	**appendix**	apéndice
teeth	dientes	**rectum**	recto
neck	cuello	**bladder**	vejiga
arm	brazo	**vagina**	vagina
shoulder	hombro	**cervix**	cervis
hand	la mano	**uterus**	útero (matriz)
fingers	dedos	**fallopian tubes**	las trompas, los tubos
axilla	axila	**ovaries**	ovarios
chest	pecho	**cyst**	quiste
breasts	pecho (seno)		

Present Pregnancy

Why did you come to the hospital (clinic)?
Porqué ha venido al hospital (a la clínica)?

Have you been coming to the clinics?
Ha venido a las clínicas?

How many times?
Cuántas veces?

When was the last time you came to the clinic? What date?
Cuándo fue la última vez que vinó a la cliníca? Qué fecha?

In what month of your pregnancy did you start prenatal care?
En qué mes de su embarazo vio al doctor para empezar el cuidado de maternidad?

Have you had any problems with this pregnancy?
Ha tenido algunos problemas con este embarazo?

What is you due date?
Para cuándo supone será la fecha del nacimiento de su bebè?

Have you had any bleeding?
Ha sangrado?

Have you had any infections? Of what?
Ha tenido algunas infecciones? De qué?

Have you had any hypertension?
Ha tenido alta presión de la sangre?

Have you had any swelling of the hand, face, legs?
Se le han hinchado las manos, el rostro (la cara), las piernas?

How much weight have you gained? How much do you weigh? Your normal weight.
Cuánto peso ha ganado? Cuánto pesa? Su peso normalmente?

Have you had spots in front of your eyes?
Ha tenido manchas enfrente de los ojos?

Have you had (severe) headaches? How many times in a week?
Ha tenido dolores (fuertes) de la cabeza? Cuántas veces en una semana?

Have you had difficulty breathing? Lying down? After working?
Ha tenido dificultad para respirar? al acostarse? Después de trabajar?

SPANISH PRIMER

Do you tire easily?
Se cansa facilmente?

Have you had heart palpitations?
Ha tenido problemas del corazón?

Have you had diarrhea? Constipation?
Ha tenido diarrea? Estreñimiento?

Labor and Delivery

Are you going to have a baby?
Va a tener un niño?

Are you in pain?
Tiene dolor?

What time did your pains begin?
Cuándo empezaron los dolores (las contracciones)?

What time did they become regular?
A qué hora fueron (empezaron) regulares (los dolores)?

How often were they once they became regular?
Con qué frecuencia cuando empezaron regulares?

How often are your pains?
Cada cuándo le dan los dolores?

How long do they last?
Cuánto duran?

Have you had bleeding?
Ha sangrado?

Was it pinkish or bright red?
Fue de color rosado o rojo claro?

How much? A cupful? A tablespoonful? A teaspoonful?
Cuánta sangre? Una taza? Una cucharada? Una cucharadita?

Did your membranes rupture? Has your bag of waters broken?
Se le revento la bolsa de agua? (Se le) ha roto la bolsa de agua?

What time did it break?
A qué hora se le revento?

Have you been vomiting?
Ha estado vomitando?

Have you had dysuria?
Ha tenido dolores al orinar?

294

How much water did you lose? Down the legs?
Cuánta agua perdió? Se le bajó por las piernas?

Have you felt the baby move today?
Ha sentido mover el niño?

Your cervix is not dilated.
Su cuello no está dilatado.

Instructions

Take off your clothes.
Quítese la ropa.

Take off your panties.
Quítese su ropa interior.

I am going to examine you.
Voy a examinarle.

Bend your knees.
Doble las rodillas.

Open your legs.
Abra las piernas.

Put your feet together.
Junte los pies.

Relax your body.
Descanse (relaje) el cuerpo.

Lie down on your back.
Acuéstese en su espalda. (Acuéstese boca arriba.)

Lie down on your right (left) side.
Acuéstese del lado derecho (izquierdo).

Move down on the table.
Bájese.

Your cervix is dilated to 5 centimeters.
Su cuello tiene cinco centímetros.

You are in labor. Your membranes have ruptured.
Está en trabajo de parto. Sus membranas están rojas.

The heartrate of the baby is normal.
El corazón del niño está normal.

Move.
Muévase.

You are going to stay in the hospital.
Se va a quedar en el hospital.

You may go home.
Se puede ir a casa.

You are in early labor.
Está en la primera parte del parto.

Stay at the hospital and walk for two hours.
Quédese aquí en el hospital y ande por dos horas.

Don't push.
No puje.

Breathe through your mouth.
Respire por la boca.

Push with your pains.
Puje con sus dolores.

Do you understand.
Entiende.

Congratulations. You have a baby boy (girl)!!
Felicitaciones. Es un niño (una niña)!

CESAREAN SECTION

Preoperative Diagnosis:
1. 42 week intrauterine pregnancy 2. Failed induction 3. Inability of the fetus to tolerate labor
Postoperative Diagnosis: Same
Procedure: Primary Low Transverse Cesarean Section via Pfannensteil
Surgeon:
Assistant:
Anesthesia: Epidural
Complications: None
EBL: 800 cc
Fluids: 1500 cc LR
Urine Output: 300 cc clear urine at end of the procedure
Indications: 20 yo G1P0 at 42 wks, induced for post-dates, late decels with oxytocin, maximum dilation 2 cm.
Findings: Male infant in cephalic presentation. Thick meconium with none below the cords, pediatrics present at delivery, Apgars 6/8, weight 2980 g. Normal uterus, tubes, and ovaries.

Procedures: The patient was taken to the operating room where epidural anesthesia was found to be adequate. She was then prepared and draped in the normal sterile fashion in the dorsal supine position with a leftward tilt. A Pfannensteil skin incision was then made with the scalpel and carried through to the underlying layer of fascia with the bovie. The fascia was incised in the midline and the incision extended laterally with the Mayo scissors. The superior aspect of the fascial incision was then grasped with the Kocher clamps, elevated, and the underlying rectus muscles dissected off bluntly. Attention was then turned to the inferior aspect of this incision which, in a similar fashion, was grasped with the Kocher clamps, and the rectus muscle dissected off bluntly. The rectus muscles were then separated in the midline, and the peritoneum identified, tented up, and entered sharply with the Metzenbaum scissors. The peritoneal incision was then extended superiorly and inferiorly with good visualization of the bladder. The bladder blade was then inserted and the vesicouterine peritoneum identified, grasped with the pick-ups and entered sharply with the Metzenbaum scissors. This incision was then extended laterally and the bladder flap created digitally.

The bladder blade was then reinserted and the lower uterine segment incised in a transverse fashion with the scalpel. The uterine incision was then extended laterally with the bandage scissors. The bladder blade was removed and the infant's head delivered atraumatically. The nose and mouth were suctioned with the DeLee suction trap, and the cord clamped and cut. The infant was handed off to the waiting pediatricians. Cord gases were sent.

The placenta was then removed manually, the uterus exteriorized, and cleared of all clots and debris. The uterine incision was repaired with 1-0 chromic in a running, locked fashion. A second layer of the same suture was used to obtain excellent hemostasis. The bladder flap was repaired with 3-0 vicryl in a running stitch and uterus returned to the abdomen. The gutters were cleared of all clots, and the peritoneum closed with 3-0 vicryl. The fascia was reapproximated with 0 vicryl in a running fashion. The skin was closed with staples.

The patient tolerated the procedure well. Sponge, lap and needle counts were correct times two. 2 grams of Cefotetan was given at cord clamp. The patient was taken to the recovery room in stable condition.

OP REPORTS

POSTPARTUM TUBAL LIGATION

Preoperative Diagnosis: Multiparity, desires permanent sterilization
Postoperative Diagnosis: Same
Procedure: Postpartum tubal ligation, Pomeroy method
Surgeon:
Assistant:
Anesthesia: Epidural
Complications: None
EBL: <20 cc
Fluids: 500 cc LR

Indications: 35 yo G5P4014 s/p NSVD who desires permanent sterilization. Risk/benefits of procedure discussed with patient including risk failure of 3-5/1000 with increased risk of ectopic gestation if pregnancy occurs.

Findings: Normal uterus, tubes, and ovaries

Procedure: The patient was taken to the operating room where her epidural was found to be adequate. A small transverse, infra umbilical skin incision was then made with the scalpel. The incision was carried down through the underlying fascia until the peritoneum was identified and entered. The peritoneum was noted to be free of any adhesions and the incision was then extended with the Metzenbaum scissors.

The patient's left fallopian tube was then identified, brought to the incision and grasped with a Babcock clamp. The tube was then followed out to the fimbria. The Babcock clamp was then used to grasp the tube approximately 4 cm from the cornual region. A 3 cm segment of tube was then ligated with a free tie of plain gut, and excised. Good hemostasis was noted and the tube was returned to the abdomen. The right fallopian tube was then ligated, and a 3 cm segment excised in a similar fashion. Excellent hemostasis was noted, and the tube returned to the abdomen.

The peritoneum and fascia were then closed in a single layer using 3-0 vicryl. The skin was closed in a subcuticular fashion using 3-0 vicryl on Keith needle.

The patient tolerated the procedure well. Sponge, lap and needle counts were correct times two. The patient was taken to the recovery room in stable condition.

Pathology: Segments of right and left fallopian tubes.

DILATION & CURETTAGE

Preoperative Diagnosis: 8 wk intrauterine pregnancy with incomplete abortion
Postoperative Diagnosis: same
Procedure: Suction D&C
Surgeon:
Assistant:
Anesthesia: Paracervical block, IV Fentanyl
Complications: None
EBL: 50 cc

Findings: 8 week sized anteverted uterus, moderate amounts of products of conception

Procedure: The patient was taken to the Special Procedure Room in the Gyn Clinic after a deformed gestational sac had been noted on transvaginal ultrasound. A sterile speculum was placed in patient's vagina and the cervix noted to be 1 cm dilated with products of conception present at the cervical os. The cervix and vagina were then swabbed with betadine and 2 cc of Xylocaine injected into the anterior lip of the cervix. The single tooth tenaculum was then applied to this location and 5 cc of Xylocaine then injected at 4 o'clock and 7 o'clock to produce a paracervical block.

The uterus was then gently sounded to 9 cm, and an 8 mm suction curett advanced gently to the uterine fundus. The suction device was then activated and the curett rotated to clear the uterus of the products of conception. A sharp curettage was then performed until a gritty texture was noted. The suction curett was then reintroduced to clear the uterus of all remaining products of conception. There was minimal bleeding noted and the tenaculum removed with good hemostasis noted.

The patient tolerated the procedure well. The patient was taken to the recovery area in stable condition.

Pathology: Products of conception.

OP REPORTS

LAPAROSCOPIC TUBAL LIGATION

Preoperative Diagnosis: Multiparity, desires permanent sterilization
Postoperative Diagnosis: Multiparity, desires permanent sterilization
Procedure: Laparoscopic tubal ligation with Falope rings
Surgeon:
Assistant:
Anesthesia: General endotracheal
Complications: None
EBL: 25 cc
Fluids: 1500 cc LR
Urine output: 100 cc clear urine at end of the procedure

Findings: Normal uterus, tubes and ovaries.

Technique: The patient was taken to the operating room where general anesthesia was obtained without difficulty. The patient was then examined under anesthesia and found to have a small anteverted uterus with normal adnexa. She was then placed in the dorsal lithotomy position and prepared and draped in the sterile fashion. A bivalve speculum was then placed in the patient's vagina and the anterior lip of the cervix grasped with the single toothed tenaculum. A HUMI uterine manipulator was then advanced into the uterus to provide a means to manipulate the uterus. The speculum was removed from the vagina.

Attention was then turned to the patient's abdomen where a 10 mm skin incision was made in the umbilical fold. The veres needle was carefully introduced into the peritoneal cavity at a 45 degree angle while tenting the abdominal wall. Intraperitoneal placement was confirmed by use of a water-filled syringe and drop in intraabdominal pressure with insufflation of CO_2 gas. The trocar and sleeve were then advanced without difficulty into the abdomen where intraabdominal placement was confirmed by the laparoscope. Pneumoperitoneum was obtained with 4 liters of CO_2 gas and the 10 mm trocar and sleeve were then advanced without difficulty into the abdomen where intraabdominal placement was confirmed by the laparoscope. A second skin incision was made 2 cm above the symphysis pubis in the midline. The second trocar and sleeve were then advanced under direct visualization.

A survey of the patient's pelvis and abdomen revealed entirely normal anatomy. The Falope ring applicator was then advanced through the second trocar sleeve and the patient's left Fallopian tube was identified and followed out to the fimbriated end. The ring was applied in the mid-isthmic area with a good knuckle of tube noted and good blanching at the site of application. There was no bleeding in the mesosalpinx. The Falope ring applicator was then reloaded and the patient's right tube manipulated in a similar fashion with easy application of the Falope ring.

The instruments were then removed from the patient's abdomen, and the incision repaired with 3-0 Vicryl. The HUMI was then removed from the vagina with no bleeding noted from the cervix. The patient tolerated the procedure well. Sponge, lap and needle counts were correct times two. The patient was taken to the recovery room in stable condition.

TOTAL ABDOMINAL HYSTERECTOMY

Preoperative Diagnosis: 1. Hypermenorrhea and Polymenorrhea unresponsive to medical therapy
Postoperative Diagnosis: 1. Hypermenorrhea and Polymenorrhea unresponsive to medical therapy
Procedure: Total abdominal hysterectomy and bilateral salpingo-oophorectomy
Surgeon:
Assistant:
Anesthesia: General endotracheal
Complications: None
EBL: 150 cc
Fluids: 1000 cc LR
Urine output: 200 cc clear urine at end of procedure
Findings: EUA: diffusely enlarged uterus. Operative finding: 8 x 7 cm uterus with normal tubes and
ovaries bilaterally. On opening the uterus a 2 x 2 cm pedunculated myoma was noted. Frozen section
revealed benign tissue. All specimens sent to pathology.

Procedure: The risks, benefits, indications, and alternatives of the procedure were reviewed with the
patient and informed consent was obtained. The patient was taken to the operating room with IV running
and Foley catheter in place.

The patient was place in the supine position, given general anesthesia, prepared and draped in the usual
sterile fashion. A Pfannensteil incision was made approximately 2 cm above the symphysis pubis and
extended sharply to the rectus fascia. The fascia was then incised bilaterally with the curved Mayo
scissors, and the muscles of the anterior abdominal wall were separated in the midline by sharp and blunt
dissection.

The peritoneum was grasped between two pick-ups, elevated and entered sharply with the scalpel. The
pelvis was examined with the finding noted above. An O'Connor - O'Sullivan retractor was placed into the
incision and the bowel packed away with moist laparotomy sponges. Two Pean clamps were place on the
cornua and used for retraction. The round ligaments on both sides were clamped, transected and suture
ligated with #0 Vicryl. The anterior leaf of the broad ligament was incised along the bladder reflection to
the midline from both sides. The bladder was then gently dissected off the lower uterine segment and the
cervix with a sponge stick.

The infundibulopelvic ligaments on both sides were then doubly clamped, transected and suture ligated
with #0 Vicryl. Hemostasis was visualized. The uterine arteries were skeletonized bilaterally, clamped
with Heaney clamps, transected and suture ligated with #0 Vicryl. Again, hemostasis was assured. The
uterosacral ligaments were clamped on both sides, transected, and suture ligated in a similar fashion.

The cervix and uterus were amputated with the cautery. The vaginal cuff angles were closed with figure-
of-eight stitches of #0 Vicryl and were transfixed to the ipsilateral cardinal and uterosacral ligaments. The
remainder of the vaginal cuff was closed with a series of interrupted #0 Vicryl figure-of-eights sutures.
Hemostasis was assured.

The pelvis was irrigated copiously with warmed normal saline. All laparotomy sponges and instrumen'
were removed from the abdomen. The fascia was closed with running #0 Vicryl, and hemostasis was
assured. The skin was closed with staples. Sponge, lap, needle and instrument counts were correct
two. The patient was taken to the PACU, awake and in stable condition.

OP REPORTS

VAGINAL HYSTERECTOMY

Preoperative Diagnosis: Uterine prolapse
Postoperative Diagnosis: Uterine prolapse
Procedure: Total vaginal hysterectomy
Surgeon:
Assistant:
Anesthesia: General endotracheal
Complications: None
EBL: 100 cc
Urine output: 200 cc clear urine at end of procedure
Fluids: 500 cc LR

Findings: EUA: small anteverted uterus with irregular contour. Operative findings: Small 7 x 6 cm irregularly shaped uterus, normal tubes, ovaries not well visualized.

Procedure: The risks, benefits, indications, and alternatives of the procedure were reviewed with the patient and informed consent was obtained. The patient was taken to the operating room with IV running and Foley catheter in place. The patient was placed in dorsolithotomy position, prepared and draped in the usual sterile fashion.

A weighted speculum was placed into the vagina, and the cervix grasped with a toothed tenaculum. The cervix was then injected circumferentially with 1% Xylocaine with 1:200,000 epinephrine. The cervix was then circumferentially incised with the scalpel and the bladder dissected off the pubovesical cervical fascia anteriorly with a sponge stick, and the Metzenbaum scissors. The anterior cul-de-sac was entered sharply. The same procedure was performed posteriorly and the posterior cul-de-sac entered sharply without difficulty.

At this point, a Heaney clamp was placed over the uterosacral ligaments on either side. These were then transected and suture ligated with #0 Vicryl. Hemostasis was assured. The cardinal ligaments were then clamped on both sides, transected and suture ligated in similar fashion.

The uterine arteries and the broad ligament were then serially clamped with Heaney clamps, transected and suture ligated on both sides. Excellent hemostasis was visualized. Both cornua were clamped with Heaney clamps, transected and the uterus delivered. These pedicles were then suture ligated with excellent hemostasis.

The peritoneum was closed with purse string suture of #0 Vicryl. The vaginal cuff angles were closed with figure-of-eight stitches of #0 Vicryl on both sides and transfixed to the ipsilateral cardinal and uterosacral ligaments. The remainder of the vaginal cuff was closed with figure-of-eight stitches of #0 Vicryl in interrupted fashion.

A Penrose drain was placed into the vaginal cuff between suture ligatures. All instruments were then removed from the vagina, and the patient taken out of dorsolithotomy position and awakened from general anesthesia. The patient was taken to the PACU in stable condition. Sponge, lap, needle and instrument count was correct times two.

SUBJECT INDEX

SUBJECT INDEX

SUBJECT INDEX

SUBJECT INDEX

SUBJECT INDEX

SUBJECT INDEX

DRUG INDEX

atorvastatin, 6
atropine, 222, 223, 224
Aventyl, 14, 15
azithromycin
    chancoid treatment, 136
    chlamydia treatment, 135
    gonorrhea treatment, 135
    STD prophylaxis, 143
AZT, 87
aztreonam, 278

B

β-blockers
    acute coronary syndrome treatment, 232
    chest pain treatment, 231
    heart rhythm conversion, 228, 229
    hypertension treatment, 9
    tachycardia conversion, 226, 227
bacterial susceptibility, to antibiotics, 277–282
beclomethasone, 54
Bendectin, 19
benzathine penicillin, 136
beta$_2$-agonists, 54–56
betamethasone suspension, 204
betamethasone valerate, 158
bethanechol, 157
bile acid resins, 6, 7
bisphosphonates, 163, 164
Blenoxane, 197
bleomycin, 197
breast abscess treatment, 48
Brevicon, 114
bromocriptine
    hyperprolactinemia treatment, 248
    polycystic ovarian syndrome treatment, 242
bronchodilators, 54
buprenorphine, 152, 153
bupropion
    depression treatment, 14, 15
buserelin
    endometriosis treatment, 146
    structure, 147
butoconazole, 131
butorphanol, 153
butyrophenones, 247

C

cabergoline, 248
calcitonin
    hypercalcemia treatment, 216
    osteoporosis treatment, 163, 165
calcium
    contractility decrease, 208
    osteoporosis treatment, 164

calcium channel blockers
    heart rhythm conversion, 228
    hypertension treatment, 8
    tachycardia conversion, 226, 227
calcium gluconate, 214
Calora, 159
captopril
    hyperkalemia cause, 214
    hypertension treatment, 8
carbamazepine, 99
carbonic anhydrase inhibitor, 215
carboplatin, 199
cation exchange resin, 214
CC, 242
CDDP, 199
cefazolin, 277
cefixime, 135
cefotaxime, 277, 279
cefotetan
    bacterial susceptibility, 277, 280
    bowel prep, 200
    endomyometritis treatment, 47
    pelvic inflammatory disease treatment, 134
cefoxitin, 133–134
ceftrazidime, 277
ceftriaxone
    bacterial susceptibility, 279
    chancoid treatment, 136
    gonorrhea treatment, 135
    pelvic inflammatory disease treatment, 133
    STD prophylaxis, 143
cefuroxime, 277, 279
Celestone, 204
Cenestin, 159
cephalosporins
    bacterial susceptibility, 277
    UTI treatment, 132
cephalosporins (1st gen.), 278, 279
Cervidil, 22
Chlor-Trimeton, 19, 54
chloramphenicol, 279, 280
chlorpheniramine
    asthma treatment, 54
    nausea treatment, 19
chlorpromazine, 19
cholestyramine, 6, 7
cimetidine, 247
ciprofloxacin
    bacterial susceptibility, 278, 279
    chancoid treatment, 136
    gonorrhea treatment, 135
    pelvic inflammatory disease treatment, 134
    urinary tract infection treatment, 132

DRUG INDEX

DRUG INDEX

DNA intercalators, 211
dobutamine, 208
dopamine
  cardiac life support, 224
  contractility decrease, 208
  ovarian hyperstimulation syndrome management, 267
dopamine agonists, 242
doxepin, 15, 16
doxorubicin
  chemotherapy characteristics, 197
  extravasation injury, 211
doxycycline
  chlamydia treatment, 135
  gonorrhea treatment, 135
  pelvic inflammatory disease treatment, 133–134
  STD prophylaxis, 143
doxylamine succinate, 19
Dramamine, 19
droperidol, 19
d4T, 87
DTIC, 199

E

efavirenz, 87
Elavil, 15, 16
enalapril, 9
Endep, 15, 16
Enoxapin, 78
epinephrine
  cardiac life support, 219, 220, 221, 222, 223, 224
  contractility decrease, 208
  neonatal resuscitation, 50
epipodophyllotoxins, 211
Epivir, 87
ergotamine, 181
erythromycin
  bacterial susceptibility, 279
  breast abscess treatment, 48
  chancroid treatment, 136
  chlamydia treatment, 135
  STD prophylaxis, 143
  Streptococcus treatment, 45
erythromycin ethylsuccinate, 135
Esclim, 159
esterified estrogens, 159
Estrace, 159
Estraderm, 159
estradiol
  dysfunctional uterine bleeding (DUB), 128
  osteoporosis treatment, 163
  ovulation induction, 256
Estratab, 159
Estratest, 159
Estring, 159

estrogen
  contraceptive use, 114
  osteoporosis treatment, 163, 164
  stress incontinence treatment, 156
estropipate, 159
Estrostep, 115
ethacrynic acid, 208
ethambutol, 280
ethinyl estradiol
  bleeding treatment, 120, 121
  contraceptive features, 114
  HRT composition, 159
  post-coital contraception, 119
ethynodiol diacetate
  contraceptive features, 114
  selection guidelines, 116–118
etidronate, 165
etoposide
  chemotherapy characteristics, 198
  extravasation injury, 211
etretinate, 100
Eurax, 158
Evista, 163, 165
Evivelle, 159

F

famciclovir, 135
Fem HRT, 159
fenofibrate, 6
fenoprofen, 153
fentanyl, 152
fibrates, 6, 7
finasteride, 245
Flagyl. see metronidazole
flecainide, 227
flouride, 165
fluoxetine
  depression treatment, 14, 15
  hot flash treatment, 181
flutamide, 245
fluvastatin, 6
folic acid antagonists, 99
Fortovase, 87
Fosamax, 163, 164
furosemide
  hypertension treatment, 9
  ovarian hyperstimulation syndrome management, 267
  preload increase, 208

G

gemcitabine, 196
gemfibrozil, 6, 7
Gemzar, 196
Genora, 114

316

DRUG INDEX

317

DRUG INDEX

DRUG INDEX

DRUG INDEX

DRUG INDEX

NOTES

NOTES

NOTES

NOTES

NOTES

NOTES

NOTES

NOTES

LABORATORY

STANFORD UNIVERSITY MEDICAL CENTER LABORATORY

Hematology

Hct	35 –47	%
Hgb	11.7-15.7	g/dL
Plt	150-400	K/uL
WBC	4.0–11.0	K/uL
Poly	42.7-73.3	%
Bands	0.0-11.0	%
Mono	2.0–11.0	%
Lymph	12.5-40.0	%
Eos	0.0-7.5	%
Baso	0.0-2.0	%
RBC	3.8-5.2	MIL/uL
MCV	82–98	fl
MCH	27–34	pg
MCHC	32–36	g/dL
RDW	11.5-14.6	%

Coagulation

PT-seconds	10.5-13.1	sec
PT-INR	0.89-1.11	INR
Coumadin range		
Low intensity	2.0-3.0	INR
High intensity	3.0-5.0	INR
APTT	23 -33	sec
Thrombin Time	13-17	sec
Fibrinogen	160-350	mg/dl
FSP	0-10	µg/mL
D-Dimer	0-200	ng/mL

Drug Levels

Carbamazepin	8-12	µg/mL
Digoxin	0.5-2.0	µg/mL
Lithium	0.6-1.2	mEq/L
Phenobarb	10-40	µg/mL
Phenytoin	10-20	µg/mL
Pro cainamide	4-8	µg/mL
Quinidine	2.5-5.0	µg/mL
Theophylline	5-20	µg/mL
Vancomycin		
Peak	20-30	µg/mL
Trough	5-10	µg/mL
Gentamycin		
Peak	6-8	ng/mL
Trough	< 2	ng/mL

Chemistry

Sodium	135-148	mEq/L
Potassium	3.5-5.3	mEq/L
Chloride	95-105	mEq/L
CO_2	24-31	mEq/L
Anion Gap	8-16	mEq/L
Osm (serum)	285-310	mOsm/kg
Glucose	70-110	mg/dL
BUN	5-25	mg/dL
Creatinine	0.5-1.4	mg/dL
Calcium	8.4-10.2	mg/dL
Calcium (ionized)	1.12-1.32	mmol/L
Phosphorous	2.5-4.5	mg/dL
Magnesium	1.5-2.0	mEq/L
Uric Acid	2.5-7.5	mg/dL
Total Protein	6.3-8.2	g/dL
Albumin	3.9-5.0	g/dL
Bilirubin, Total	0.2-1.3	mg/dL
Bilirubin, Direct	0.0-0.4	mg/dL
Alk Phos	38-126	IU/L
AST (SOOT)	8-39	IU/L
ALT (SGPT)	9-52	IU/L
Gamma GT	8-78	IU/L
Cholesterol		
Low Risk	< 200	mg/dL
Moderate Risk	200-239	mg/dL
High Risk	> 239	mg/dL
Triglyceride	35-135	mg/dL
Amylase	30-110	IU/L
Ammonia	9-33	µmol/L
Ferritin		
Female 18-50 yo	6-81	ng/mL
Female > 50 yo	14-186	ng/mL
Male	30-284	ng/mL
Iron		
Female	37-170	µg/dL
Male	49-181	µg/dL
TIBC	250-450	%
Transferrin	230-430	mg/dL
Haptoglobin	50-320	mg/dL

LABORATORY

ENDOCRINE LAB VALUES

	Conventional Units	Conversion Factor	SI Units
ACTH, adrenocorticotropin hormone			
6:00 AM	10-80 pg/mL	0.2202	2.2-17.6 pmol/L
6:00 PM	<50 pg/mL	0.2202	<11 pmol/L
Androstenedione	60-300 ng dL	0.0349	2.1-10.5 nmol/L
Cortisol			
8:00 AM	5-25 μg/dL	27.9	140-700 nmol/L
4:00 PM	3-12 μg/dL	27.9	80-330 nmol/L
10:00 PM	<50% of AM value	27.9	<50% of AM value
Dehydroepiandrosterone sulfate	80-350 μg/dL	0.0027	2.2-9.5 μmol/L
11-Deoxycortisol	0.05-0.25 μg/dL	28.86	1.5-7.3 nmol/L
11-Deoxycorticosterone	2-10 ng/dL	30.3	60-300 pmol/l
Estradiol	20-400 pg/mL	3.67	70-1500 pmol/L
Estrone	30-200 pg/mL	3.7	110-740 pmol/L
FSH, reproductive years	5-30 mIU/mL	1.0	5-30 IU/L
Glucose, fasting	70-110 mg/dL	0.0556	4.0-6.0 mmol/L
Growth hormone	<10 ng/mL	1.0	<10 μg/L
17-Hydroxyprogesterone	100-300 ng/dL	0.03	3-9 nmol/L
Insulin, fasting	5-25 μU/mL	7.175	35-180 pmol/L
Insulin-like growth factor-1	0.3-2.2 U/mL	1000	300-2200 U/L
LH, reproductive years	5-20 mIU/mL	1.0	5-20 IU/L
Progesterone			
Follicular phase	<3 ng/mL	3.18	<9.5 nmol/L
Secretory phase	5-30 ng/mL	3.18	16-95 nmol/L
Prolactin	1-20 ng/mL	44.4	44.4-888 pmol/L
Testosterone, total	20-80 ng/dL	0.0347	0.7-2.8 nmol/L
Testosterone, free	100-200 pg/mL	0.0347	35-700 pmol/L
TSH, thyroid stimulating hormone	0.35-6.7 μU/mL	1.0	0.35-6.7 mU/L
Thyroxine, free T4	0.8-2.3 ng/dL	1.29	10-30 nmol/L
Triiodothyronine, T3, total	80-220 ng/dL	0.0154	1.2-3.4 nmol/L
Triidothyronine, T3, free	0.13-0.55 ng/dL	15.4	2.0-8.5 pmol/L
Triiodothyronine, reverse	8-35 ng/dL	15.4	120-540 pmol/L

Source: Speroff L, Glass RH, Kase NG. Clinical Assays. In: *Clinical Gynecologic Endocrinology and Infertility.* 5th ed. Baltimore: Williams & Wilkins, 1994. Reproduced with the permission of the publisher.